PACIFIC PARK

D0939444

TRUSTING BIRTH
WITH THE BONAPACE METHOD

English Translation: Megan Millward
Proofreading : Camalo Gaskin
Graphic design: Editorial Sirio, S.A.
Photography: Tango
Infography: Nicole Lafond
Scanner operator: Mélanie Sabourin

Catalogue data available from Bibliothèque
et Archives nationales du Québec

EXCLUSIVE DISTRIBUTORS:

For Canada and the United States:
MESSAGERIES ADP*
2315, De la Province St.
Longueuil, Québec J4G 1G4
Tél.: 450-640-1237
Fax: 450-674-6237
Internet : www.messageries-adp.com
* subsidiary of the Sogides Group Inc.,
  a subsidiary of Québecor Média Inc.

For France and other countries:
INTERFORUM editis
Immeuble Paryseine,
3 Allée de la Seine
94854 Ivry Cedex
Tél.: 01 49 59 11 56/91
Fax: 01 49 59 11 33
Orders:
Tél.: 02 38 32 71 00
Fax: 02 38 32 71 28

For Switzerland:
INTERFORUM editis SWITZERLAND
P.O. Box 69 - 1701 Fribourg - Switzerland
Tél.: (41-26) 460-80-60
Fax: (41-26) 460-80-68
Internet : www.havas.ch
E-mail : office@havas.ch
Distribution : OLF SA
Z.I. 3, Corminbœuf
P.O. Box 1061
CH-1701 Fribourg
Orders :
Tél.: (41-26) 467-53-33
Fax: (41-26) 467-54-66

For Belgium and Luxembourg :
INTERFORUM BENELUX S.A.
Fond Jean-Pâques, 6
B-1348 Louvain-La-Neuve
Téléphone : 32 (0) 10 42 03 20
Fax : 32 (0) 10 41 20 24
Internet : www.interforum.be
Courriel : info@interforum.be

07-15

© 2008, Juniper Publishing,
division of the Sogides Group Inc.,
a subsidiary of Québecor Média Inc.
(Montreal, Quebec)

Legal deposit: 2015
National Library of Québec
National Library of Canada

ISBN 978-1-988002-17-0

Conseil des Arts   Canada Council
du Canada   for the Arts

We gratefully acknowledge the support of the Canada Council
for the Arts for its publishing program.

We acknowledge the financial support of the Government of
Canada through the Book Publishing Industry Development
Program (BPIDP) for our publishing activities.

JULIE BONAPACE

TRUSTING BIRTH
WITH THE BONAPACE METHOD
Keys to Loving your Birth Experience

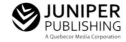

JUNIPER
PUBLISHING
A Quebecor Media Corporation

*For my daughter Malika, my mother Marie, and my partner Lawrence
for their support and unconditional love*

PREFACE

Julie Bonapace has created an innovative pain management and birth preparation method. Since 1989 she has been teaching this method, which has become well-known around the world. In keeping with the recommendations of the World Health Organization (WHO) and the ministries of health of various countries, she presents pregnancy and birth as an important human experience, whose natural character should be maintained while benefiting from scientific progress.

Bonapace has developed this method to make labor easier and birth more pleasant for mothers. Her interest is also to promote the active involvement of the father in this stage of life, so that he is present, feels attached to his child and implicated in the child's development. The perinatal period remains a crucial stage in the creation and development of attachment between the child and its mother and father.

It is with great pride that the University of Montreal Hospital Center has been teaching the *Bonapace Method* at the Saint-Luc Hospital since 2000. Each year, couples benefit from training as well as structured support, under the leadership of our nurse, Johanne Steben, who was trained in what we see as an excellent birth preparation method.

Our clinicians, nurses and doctors, recognize that women who give birth using the *Bonapace Method* better understand the process of birth, are more relaxed, and manage pain more efficiently.

We have noticed that partners involved in the process participate more actively in the birth of their child. They do not seem disconcerted, and frequently feel useful and proud of their contribution to this joyous event, especially because their help is so central in their partner's management of pain.

We have also seen that effective companionship during the birth allows for a reduction in obstetrical interventions such as epidurals, instrument-assisted births, and cesarean sections.

All of our clinicians highly recommend that couples learn the *Bonapace Method* for the management of the wonderful but nerve-wracking adventure that is the birth of their child.

MARIE-JOSÉE BÉDARD, M.D., F.R.C.S. (C)
Chief of Obstetrics and Gynecology
University of Montreal Hospital Center

FOREWORD

It is with great delight that I share with you the fruits of a nearly two-year long 'pregnancy': the English edition of *Trusting Birth with the Bonapace Method*. Grounded in new scientific evidence, as well as the wisdom of women, their partners, researchers, midwives, doctors and doulas from all over the world, this new edition presents many tools to help you give birth in a relaxed, safe, and satisfying manner.

This method is at its essence a practical process. It is centered on establishing practices that you rely on throughout your pregnancy and birth. In the process of pregnancy and birth these will serve to benefit you during your most intense moments. It is a method based on research I worked on in the University of Quebec's Pain Management Laboratory, where we investigated non-pharmacological pain management. This method was also borne out of my own research into tools for creating a 'zen state' to cope with life's intense situations.

Through practice, knowledge becomes skill. For this reason, this book does not primarily focus on *what* occurs in birth but on *how* to allow birth to occur by establishing practices that enable you to activate your innate neurophysiological resources (chapter 2). It recommends that you physically prepare for the birth by creating a practice of yoga poses (asanas), breathing, movement and massage (chapters 1, 4, 5, and 6). To support the physiological mechanisms that greatly benefit us in birth, preparation requires an understanding of *how* to respect and rely on your body's innate hormonal functions (chapter 3). In the following pages you will find all the information needed to work with the different mechanisms at play during labor and birth. This knowledge will help you establish a fundamental trust that women's bodies have everything that is needed to give birth to a healthy child.

The book presents practical exercises, including relaxation and mental imagery (chapters 7 and 8), that support you in developing a positive attitude throughout your pregnancy and childbirth experience. Watching the recommended films will also help to anchor these notions in your imagination. Finally, the book illustrates how practicing the Emotional Freedom Technique (EFT) will support you in coping with those intense and difficult moments within your pregnancy and birth.

The approach that I share is steeped in scientific research. It sometimes calls into question certain practices that are still common during childbirth. Ingrained habits can be difficult to change in institutional settings like hospitals. For this reason, it is important that you be informed and determined to make adequate preparations to have your choices respected. Surround yourself with people who support your birth plan. Carefully choose a place to birth and healthcare professionals who will accompany you over the course of your pregnancy and birth. Prepare your wishes for the birth and discuss them with your providers. You will notice that I've chosen to replace some words or expressions that may have a negative connotation by more empowering and positive words. For example, contractions are referred to as rushes, false labor as preliminary labor and pain as sensations.

The preparation described in this book includes your partner and gives them an active role in the foreground. This offers you, as a couple, the opportunity to experience the birth of your family together. It also enables mothers and their partners to each develop the skills and competences needed to confront the intense situations they may encounter during pregnancy and birth.

Playing an important role during this period affirms the importance of your partner in the family. Studies show that fathers who prepare themselves for the birth of their child and who know how to support a woman in labor participate more in the care of the baby during the postnatal period than do fathers who were not prepared[1]. Involvement reinforces their self-esteem. Father-mother and father-child relationships are also made stronger.

The better the relationship between the couple, the stronger the father-child bond[2]. Satisfaction of both partners is greater and the passage into the parental role occurs with more ease[3].

My work as family mediator, responsible for negotiating divorces, convinced me of the importance of including the partner in the preparation for birth. If, however, your partner will not be participating in the birth of your child, do not hesitate to find a support person (e.g. doula, family member, or friend) who will know how to provide continuous support during the course of labor and birth. With all my heart, I wish you a journey filled with discoveries and a safe, relaxed and satisfying birth.

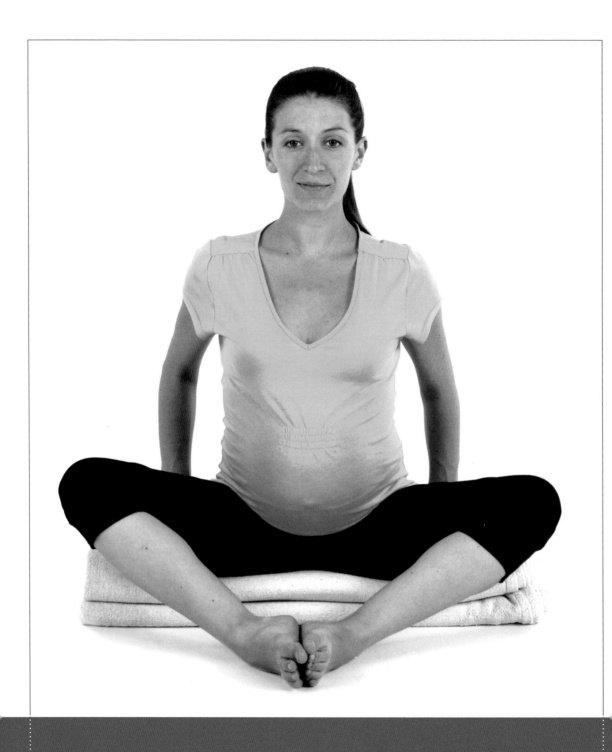

Chapter 1

PREPARATION

A proverb has long reminded us that *it is better to prevent than to cure.* This is exactly what the Bonapace Method suggests for the prenatal period. Being in good physical shape helps to create conditions that ease the birthing process. Since women give birth with their bodies, it is important for their body to be strong, supple and well-aligned. To guide you in attaining this goal, this method recommends that you practice a yoga routine that includes poses (asanas)[4] that will target the areas of the body that are most needed during pregnancy: the chest, the lower back, the abdominal muscles, legs, adductors (inner thigh muscles), the pelvic floor and the piriformis (buttocks) muscle. Besides helping you to relax, this yoga routine, when practiced regularly, will allow your baby to get into the optimal position in your womb, that is, head down, and back facing forward.

It is not necessary for you to be accustomed to yoga to appreciate the benefits of the routine that is presented in this chapter. The movements are simple and clearly illustrated, in order to facilitate your daily practice, no matter which stage of pregnancy you're in. I encourage you to make good use of this period to be in touch with your baby; it is an excellent moment for bonding. Observe your baby's movements and pay attention to the sensations while you are in the poses.

To ease certain discomforts of pregnancy such as back pain, constipation, cramping in your calves, etc, use massage and adapted poses that will help you to minimize medical interventions. For example, practicing perineal massage reduces injuries in that area, and the practice of certain yoga poses strengthens the body and makes it more flexible. This allows you to give birth in a variety of positions.

Summary of Chapter 1: Preparation

OBJECTIVE	METHOD
Promote mother and baby's well-being during the pregnancy	• Practice appropriate poses (seated, standing, lying down) • Practice yoga daily to relax and reduce stress • Communicate mentally and emotionally with baby
Promote a physiological and stress-free birth	• Practice yoga to strengthen and relax the body • Practice yoga and poses to promote optimal positioning of baby in the uterus
Become aware of one's body	• Practice yoga
Relieve back pain and body tension	• Practice correct posture in daily life • Practice yoga • Massage the piriformis muscle
Prevent injury to the perineum	• Practice yoga • Massage the perineum

During the weeks preparing for birth, I encourage you to prepare physically for the birth by dedicating yourself to daily yoga practice, by maintaining correct posture when standing, sitting, and lying down, and by massaging certain parts of your body.

As the partner, your role lies in supporting the pregnant woman in her regular piriformis (buttocks) massage and perineal massage, as well as in preparing to work together with her during pregnancy and birth.

YOGA DURING PREGNANCY

Pregnancy changes a woman's body. The increase in weight and the secretion of a hormone called relaxin have an effect on muscles and tissues. The body's elasticity increases, and its capacity to react to stress changes. All these phenomena justify the importance of developing good habits to prepare yourself for birth.

Yoga is a science as well as an art that dates back thousands of years. It is a discipline available to everyone. Regular practice allows you to benefit in the present moment. Attention is given to your sensations, and your breath accompanies your movements. Yoga calms the mind and puts it in harmony with the body. This produces a better physical, mental and spiritual harmony whenever you put it into practice.

There are many types of yoga. The one featured in this book is hatha yoga as it was taught by B.K.S. Iyengar[5], a yogi who started teaching yoga in 1936, at the age of 18. He brilliantly adapted the practice of poses so that "the young, the aged, the weak and the sick" could also benefit from them. This type of yoga respects your body's limitations by introducing supports (blocks, straps, blankets, walls, chairs, etc) to help you achieve poses that might otherwise be difficult during pregnancy. Iyengar yoga focuses on body alignment, symmetry, and the pursuit of precision in poses. Besides developing flexibility, strength, and endurance, practicing asanas (poses) allows you to improve your ability to concentrate and to relax, in other words, your ability to enter a 'zen state', which will be very useful to you during birth.

The Benefits of Yoga

Establishing a prenatal yoga practice has been part of the Bonapace Method since 1989. Before prenatal yoga practice was a common option for pregnant women, as it is today, this resource was under-utilized. I studied the benefits and taught these principles and postures as the foundational practices of the early Bonapace Method. In the last decade prenatal yoga has really caught on as a popular practice in preparing women for childbirth. Recent studies also show the benefits of yoga for prenatal preparation. In the field of medicine, the most robust and highly respected studies are randomized controlled studies. In my own research, I have relied mostly on these studies to help many women better understand the benefits of the practices I recommend. One such study revealed that six hours of yoga training coupled with practicing poses (asanas) and breathing (pranayama) three times a week, starting from the 26th week of pregnancy, improve maternal well-being during labor, birth, and the first two hours post-partum (after birth). These practices reduce the perception of pain and reduce the total length of labor and birth[6].

Another study compared women who practiced yoga an hour a day starting from the 20th week of pregnancy with women who walked for 30 minutes twice a day starting at the same stage of pregnancy. The women from the yoga group had been to four or five training sessions with a qualified instructor. Among the women practicing yoga there was a reduction in the number of premature births, fewer low-birth-weight babies (5.5 lbs. 2500 g, or less), less isolated intra-uterine growth retardation (IUGR) and less pregnancy-induced hypertension with associated IUGR. No side effects were reported[7].

As you can see, these are wonderful benefits for a non-invasive approach that only requires a few hours of practice per week! The advantage of this technique is to allow you to really live in your body. You learn to work with your body as a resource. Ultimately, you give birth with your body, not with your mind. The yogi K. Pattabhi Jois summed up this concept well when he said that yoga is 99% practice and 1% theory[8].

Certain parts of a pregnant woman's body are called upon more than others during pregnancy and birth. The yoga practice that I recommend at the end of this chapter prepares the body for birth by targeting these particular areas.

The poses described have multiple benefits:

- They relax the paravertebral muscles, especially those of the lower back that ensure good upright posture (these muscles protect against the forward-movement of the pelvis caused by the weight of the baby).
- They tone and relax the muscles of the adductors (inner thighs) and those of the perineum (pelvic floor). When these muscles are strong they help ensure good support and stability of the pelvic bones. Flexible muscles allow for the extraordinary opening of the pelvis and the passage of the baby during birth.
- They help you become aware of the deep perineum in order to be better able to relax it during birth.
- They tone the deep abdominal muscles that will contribute to maintaining good posture.
- They increase flexibility in your piriformis (buttocks) muscle, which is attached to the sacrum and is often tense. In many cases, this tension leads to pains that radiate to the buttocks, hips and thighs.

Some Basic Principles of Yoga Practice

Here are some basic concepts to keep in mind during your yoga practice. They will also help ensure your well-being and that of your child:

- Yoga is to be practiced gently, with respect for your body. Pay attention to your sensations, and make gradual progress. The key is regular practice.
- Breath should be harmonious, silent, and effortless. It is always free, never blocked. Let your whole body breathe.
- If your breathing is short, tight, or forced, it is a sign that your pose is incorrect. Start the pose again, elongating your back and releasing your shoulders.
- In between poses, rest as needed by lying down on your side.
- Stop any movement that causes pain or any type of discomfort.
- After each supine pose, roll onto your side and come to a seated position before standing up.
- If you need help, contact a qualified instructor.

STANDING POSES

As her baby develops, a pregnant woman will tend to lean her upper body back. She arches her back to maintain her balance, which increases pressure on the interior of the abdomen, against the abdominal muscles (rectus abdominis muscles) and the perineal muscles. To maintain correct upright posture, I recommend that you always lengthen your back by lifting your chest and slightly lowering the tailbone.

BASIC STANDING POSE –*Tadasana*

The Tadasana pose is one of yoga's most fundamental poses; its name means "stable and straight like a mountain". The pressure under the feet is spread evenly between three points: the bottom of the big toe, the bottom of the little toe, and the bottom of the heel (*illustration 1.1*). Move back and forth to find the point of equilibrium at the center of the sole of your feet. During the third trimester, you will need to turn your big toes slightly in-wards in order to make space in your lower back.

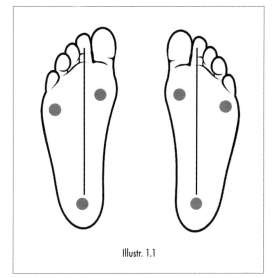

Illustr. 1.1

STEPS

1. Stand upright, with your feet hip-width apart (*figure 1.1*).
2. Feet flat on the floor, weight evenly distributed among the three points of the feet.
3. Lengthen your toes without tensing them.
4. Feet are parallel and heels are in line with each other.
5. Stretch and lift the kneecaps by firming the quadriceps (thigh muscles).
6. Roll the thighs from the outside inwards to release the sacrum (the bone at the base of your spine).
7. Point the sacrum toward the floor. Keep the sacrum in a neutral position, not arched back or tucked under.
8. Lift your belly and gently tuck the lower ribs in.
9. Lengthen your spine and lift the chest.
10. Open the shoulders and chest by lifting the arms on either side of the body, palms to the sky.

11. Drop the shoulder blades, turn your palms and lower your arms so that they are alongside your body (*figure 1.2*).

12. Your head and neck are straight. Face and eyes are soft (*figure 1.3*).

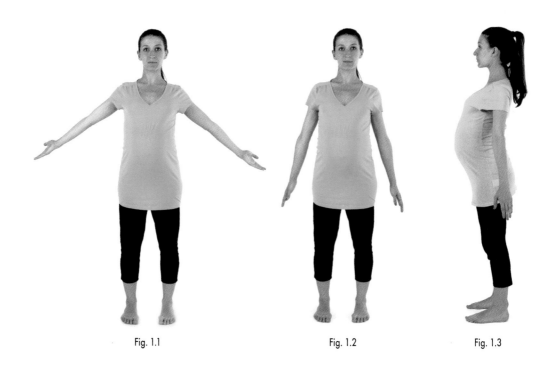

Fig. 1.1   Fig. 1.2   Fig. 1.3

Beneficial Effects

- Prevents back pain linked to arching of the lower back.
- Promotes pelvic alignment so that the baby gets into optimal position.
- Relieves leg cramps at night.

At the end of the pregnancy, you may feel an uncomfortable weight at the bottom of the vagina or behind the pubic bone. This unpleasant sensation may cause you to want to close your pelvis by crossing your legs and tightening your buttocks, which creates involuntary muscle contractions and tension in the deep perineum. To correct this heaviness and maintain correct upright posture, train yourself to stand up straight.

STANDING POSE WITH SUPPORTED FOOT

When you need to stay standing for an extended period of time, wear flat shoes or low heels that support your feet well, and place a stool under one foot. Avoid asymmetry of the hips by keeping the foot on the floor aligned with the knee and hip.

STANDING POSE WITH LEG TO THE SIDE – *Marichyasana 1*

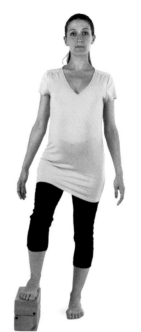

Fig. 1.4

STEPS

1. Place a chair next to you and another in front of you.
2. Stand in standing pose (*figure 1.2*) with one chair touching the side of your leg.

   ◆ Stand upright, with your feet hip-width apart (*figure 1.1*).
   ◆ Feet flat on the floor, weight evenly distributed among the three points of the feet.
   ◆ Lengthen your toes without tensing them.
   ◆ Feet are parallel and heels are in line with one another.
   ◆ Stretch and lift the kneecaps by firming the quadriceps (thigh muscles).
   ◆ Roll the thighs from the outside inwards to release the sacrum (the bone at the base of your spine).
   ◆ Point the sacrum toward the floor. Keep the sacrum in a neutral position, not arched back or tucked under.
   ◆ Lift your belly and gently tuck the lower ribs in.
   ◆ Lengthen your spine and lift the chest.
   ◆ Open the shoulders and chest by lifting the arms on either side of the body, palms to the sky.
   ◆ Lower the shoulder blades, turn your palms and lower your arms so that they are alongside your body (*figure 1.2*).
   ◆ Your head and neck are straight. Face and eyes are soft (*figure 1.3*).

3. Lift the leg next to the chair and place the foot at a 45 degree angle in the center of the chair.

4. The foot of the standing leg is straight, with the ankle, hip, and knee aligned with each other.
5. Lower the hip of the bent leg so that both hips are at the same height.
6. Breathe in this position for a few moments.
7. Place your hands in the hollow of the groin and bend forward as you lengthen the back and lift the chest.
8. Place your hands on the seat of the chair in front of you, lengthen the head, the neck, and back. Gently tuck the lower ribs in and lift the chest (*figure 1.5*).
9. Breathe in this position for a few seconds.
10. To come out of the pose, place your hand on the bent knee. By supporting yourself on the knee, come up keeping your back straight.

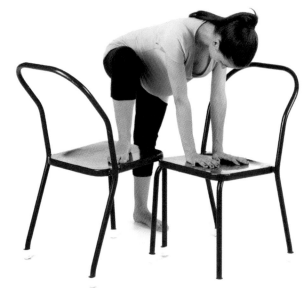

Fig. 1.5

11. With the opposite hand, lift the leg and place it on the floor.
12. Come back to the standing pose (Tadasana).

PLEASE ENSURE THAT:
- The chest is lifted and the back is lengthened.
- The kneecap of the standing leg is lifted, the thigh muscles are firm.
- The hips are horizontal.

Beneficial Effects:
- ◆ Relieves pain of the back, shoulders, neck and sacro-iliac joints (lower back).
- ◆ Increases pelvic flexibility.
- ◆ Tones the abdominal muscles.

Caution or Special Support

The more your pregnancy progresses, the more distance there should be between the legs.

SEATED POSES

To prevent back pain and aid digestion and breathing in a seated position, always lengthen the back and open the chest.

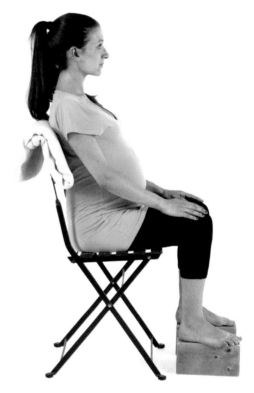

Fig. 1.6

SEATED POSE ON A CHAIR

STEPS

1. Place the feet on the floor, hip-width apart. The knees are at the same level as the hips. If the chair is too high, put your feet on blankets, books, or blocks (*figure 1.6*).
2. The leg bones are parallel to each other and to the floor.
3. Do not round the back. Try rather to lengthen it by gently tucking in the lower ribs, lifting the chest, and rolling the shoulders back while lowering them. Place a blanket behind your back, in order to support the shoulder blades.
4. Sit on the center of your ischia (the pointed bones under the buttocks).
5. Rise from the chair by leaning your upper body forward, with your back straight[9].
6. Exhale while pressing your legs or pressing against the arms of the chair.

SEATED POSE ON A CHAIR, SUPPORTED BY A WALL

This posture can be practiced at any time throughout pregnancy. It works to relax tensions in the upper body. In active labor, the chair can be replaced by a ball.

STEPS

1. Place the seat of a chair facing a wall.
2. Sit on the edge of the chair. While straddling the chair, your legs should be far enough apart that the space underneath your belly is free. Your toes should touch the wall with your knees above your feet.
3. Slide your hands up the wall as you exhale. Your arms should be slightly more than shoulder-width apart (*figure 1.7*).
4. Your back should be lengthened and your lower ribs are slightly back.

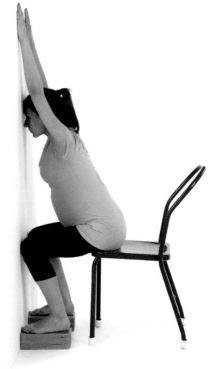

Fig. 1.7

> **PLEASE ENSURE THAT:**
> • The lower back is not over-arching.
> • The sacrum is lengthened toward the floor.

SEATED POSE SUPPORTED BY A WALL - *Utkatasana*

This pose strengthens the legs, which are particularly called upon during the bearing down and birthing stage of labor.

STEPS

1. Come into the standing position (*figure 1.2*) about 12 inches (30 cm) away from the wall, back to the wall.

   ◆ Stand upright, with your feet hip-width apart (*figure 1.1*).
   ◆ Feet flat on the floor, weight evenly distributed among the three points of the feet.
   ◆ Lengthen your toes without tensing them.
   ◆ Feet are parallel and heels are in line with one another.
   ◆ Stretch and lift the kneecaps by firming the quadriceps (thigh muscles).
   ◆ Roll the thighs from the outside inwards to release the sacrum (the bone at the base of your spine).

- Point the sacrum toward the floor. Keep the sacrum in a neutral position, not arched back or tucked under.
- Lift your belly and gently tuck the lower ribs in.
- Lengthen your spine and lift the chest.
- Open your shoulders and chest by lifting the arms on either side of the body, palms to the sky.
- Lower your shoulder blades, turn your palms and lower your arms so that they are alongside your body (*figure 1.2*).
- Your head and neck are straight. Face and eyes are soft (*figure 1.3*).

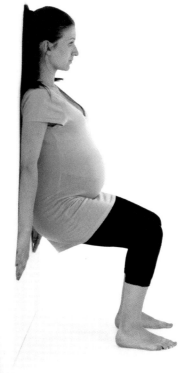

Fig. 1.8

2. Press your fingertips against the wall behind you, then press your back against the wall.
3. Keeping the back lengthened, breathe while bending your knees and letting your buttocks slide downward (*figure 1.8*).
4. Keep the pose for 15 - 30 seconds. Adjust according to your capacity.
5. To come out of the pose, inhale as you straighten your legs to return to the starting position.

PLEASE ENSURE THAT:
- Your back is straight and supported against the wall. It is lengthened and in contact with the wall.
- Your buttocks slide down toward the floor without leaving the wall.
- Your upper body maintains the standing posture (*figure 1.2*).

Beneficial Effects:
- Tones your back and abdominal muscles.
- Strengthens your leg muscles.
- Increases ankle, knee and leg flexibility.

This pose is the starting point for seated poses.

STEPS

1. Sit on a stack of three or four blankets, so that your buttocks are higher than your feet.
2. Make sure you are sitting straight, with your legs out in front of you, feet apart, extending through the heels to stretch the legs (*figure 1.9*).
3. Lengthen your toes toward the ceiling.
4. Keep the palms of your hands faced down next to your hips, with the fingers pointing toward your legs.

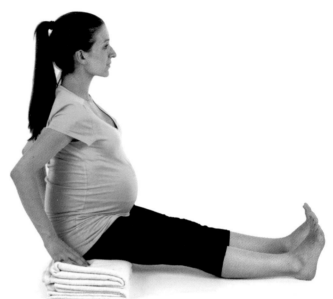

Fig. 1.9

5. Lift your belly and press your thighs (femur bones) against the floor, extending through the heels to stretch the legs.
6. Lengthen the spine and lift the chest by bringing your elbows closer together, slightly behind you.
7. Your head and neck are straight. Face and eyes are soft.
8. Stay in this pose from 30 to 60 seconds, breathing softly.

Beneficial Effects:

- Stretches your leg muscles.
- Massages your abdominal muscles.
- Strengthens the muscles around your spine.
- Tones your kidneys.

Caution or Special Support

If you have a weak back or if you suffer from cardiac problems, support your back against a wall.

SEATED POSE – *Svastikasana*

This is an excellent pose to practice when you are seated on the floor. The supports placed under the buttocks facilitate getting into the position, and prevent your respiratory diaphragm and your lungs from becoming compressed by a rounded back. This enables you to take full inhalations and exhalations.

STEPS

1. Start with the seated pose, legs extended (*figure 1.9*).

    - Sit on a stack of three or four blankets, so that your buttocks are higher than your feet.
    - Make sure you are sitting straight, with your legs out in front of you, feet apart (*figure 1.9*).
    - Lengthen your toes toward the ceiling.
    - Keep the palms of your hands facing down next to your hips, with the fingers pointing toward your legs.
    - Lift your belly and gently tuck the lower ribs in.
    - Lengthen your spine and lift your chest by bringing your elbows closer together.
    - Your head and neck are straight. Face and eyes are soft.

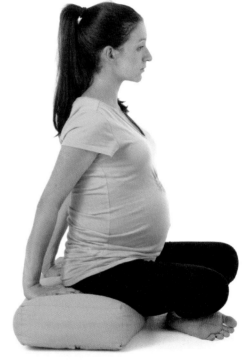

Fig. 1.10

2. Bend the right knee outward and place the right foot under the left thigh.

3. Bend the left knee outward and place the left foot under the right thigh (*figure 1.10*).
4. Your shin bones (tibias) should be crossed in the middle. Each foot is placed under the opposite knee.
5. Open the chest by placing the hands facing downward to each side of the hips. Fingers facing forward toward your legs. Bring your elbows toward one another, lower the shoulders and bring your shoulder blades together.
6. Without moving the upper body, place the tops of your hands on your thighs, near the groin.

Beneficial Effects:
- Releases your pelvis and back.
- Facilitates better breathing.

> **PLEASE ENSURE THAT:**
> - Your spine is firm and centered.
> - Your abdominal organs are lifted.

Caution or Special Support
As needed, press yourself against the wall for more support.

SEATED POSE WITH LEGS IN BUTTERFLY POSITION - *Badha Konasana*

This pose is one that I most highly recommend for pregnant women, due to its effect on your kidneys, pelvic floor, and your breathing. Use a support under your buttocks so that you can lift the spine without overworking the lower back.

STEPS
1. Start with the seated pose, legs extended (*figure 1.9*)

- Sit on a stack of three or four blankets, so that your buttocks are higher than your feet.
- Make sure you are sitting straight, with your legs out in front of you, feet apart (*figure 1.9*).
- Lengthen your toes toward the ceiling.
- Keep the palms of your hands facing down next to your hips, with the fingers pointing toward your legs.
- Lift your belly and gently tuck the lower ribs in.
- Lengthen your spine and lift the chest by bringing your elbows closer together.
- Your head and neck are straight. Face and eyes are soft.

2. Bend both legs at the knees and pull your feet toward the groin (*figure 1.11*).
3. Bring your soles and heels of your feet together so that they touch.
4. Hold the feet with your hands or with a strap, and bring the heels toward the perineum. The outer edges of the feet should be in contact with the floor. Breathe normally.
5. Expand your thighs gently moving the knees toward the floor.
6. Hold the pose for 5 to 6 minutes, breathing softly.

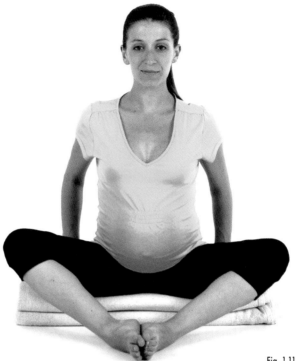

Fig. 1.11

Beneficial Effects:

- Relieves back pain and strengthens your pelvic and lower back muscles.
- Creates space in the birth canal and stretches your pelvic floor muscles.
- Relieves the feeling of heaviness in your pelvis and facilitates breathing.

Caution or Special Support

If you feel discomfort around the pubic bone, add more height with blankets and make sure you have support under your thighs.

SEATED POSE, LEGS APART - *Upavishta Konasana*

In this pose, the legs are apart in order to create an angle between the two legs that varies between 90 and 180 degrees. As in the preceding pose, the goal is to strengthen, open and make the pelvis more flexible. At birth, a considerable amount of pressure will be put on the pelvic joints. When you are strong and flexible, you can better work with the intense sensations of the bearing down and birthing stage.

STEPS

1. Start with the seated pose, legs extended (*figure 1.9*)

   ◆ Sit on a stack of three or four blankets, so that your buttocks are higher than your feet.
   ◆ Make sure you are sitting straight, with your legs out in front of you, feet apart.
   ◆ Lengthen your toes toward the ceiling.
   ◆ Keep the palms of your hands facing down next to your hips, with the fingers pointing toward your legs.
   ◆ Lift your belly and gently tuck the lower ribs in.
   ◆ Lengthen your spine and lift your chest by bringing your elbows closer together.
   ◆ Your head and neck are straight. Face and eyes are soft.

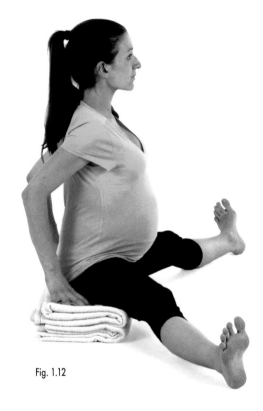

Fig. 1.12

2. Spread your legs apart by extending them outward starting at the heel, one part of the leg after the other, in order to avoid cramps. Gradually increase the angle between your legs (*figure 1.12*).

3. The soles of the feet are perpendicular to the floor and the toes point up to the ceiling. Be sure that the feet do not fall inwards.

4. Continue practicing this pose even if you feel an intense sensation in the hamstring muscles (behind the thighs). With time, this sensation will diminish.

5. Keep the palms of your hands on the floor, next to your outer thighs.

> **PLEASE ENSURE THAT:**
> • The backs of your legs move toward the floor.
> • Your legs are lengthened through the heels, despite their tendency to rise.
> • Your shoulders are rolled back to open and lift your chest. Your lower ribs are in and lifted, which increases the distance between the diaphragm and the lower part of the abdomen.

6. Lift your waist and ribs up by extending your legs through the heels and by pushing your palms against the floor.
7. Lift the chest.

Beneficial Effects:
- Strengthens your pelvic floor muscles and back muscles.
- Improves circulation in your pelvis and abdomen.
- Tones the kidneys, which helps with urinary problems.

Caution or Special Support
Avoid this pose if your baby has descended prematurely, or if your cervix has started to dilate or has ever been injured in any way. If your spine feels heavy, roll up a small towel and place it under your tailbone (or coccyx).

KNEELING POSE – *Virasana*

This pose for strength and power opens up your breathing and aligns your back.

1. Kneel on the floor, with your knees apart and your shins parallel (*figure 1.13*). To avoid pressure on the joints of the knees and ankles, place some blankets piled on top of each other under your buttocks, so that they are higher than your feet (*figure 1.14*).
2. Roll your calves outward so that your shins rest on the floor.
3. Distribute your weight between the knees, feet and buttocks.
4. Apply light pressure on the outer edges of the feet and press them toward the floor.
5. Lengthen your lower back. The sacrum points to the floor (*figure 1.15*).
6. Stretch out your upper body by lifting your waist and the sides of the chest. Your lower ribs are gently tucked in, your shoulders are rolled back and lowered toward the waist. Be careful not to overextend the lower back.
7. Place the palms of your hands on your knees or ankles.
8. Breathe normally. Keep this position for about a minute.
9. To come out of the pose, bring the weight of your upper body forward and lift yourself up onto your knees (*figure 1.16*).

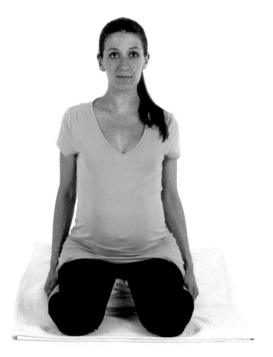

Fig. 1.13

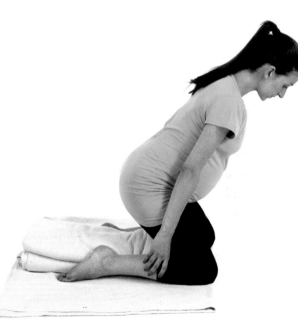

Fig. 1.14

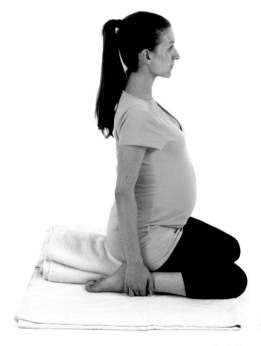

Fig. 1.15

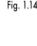

Fig. 1.16

TRUSTING BIRTH WITH THE BONAPACE METHOD

Beneficial Effects:

- Elevating your buttocks prevents slouching, and creates a lengthened, straight back which creates courage and confidence.
- Prevents and relieves swollen legs and varicose veins.
- Corrects overextension in your lower back.
- Reduces elevated arterial tension caused by kidney problems.

> **PLEASE ENSURE THAT:**
> - Your upper body is straight and not leaning forward.
> - Your thighs and groin move downwards.

Caution or Special Support

Elevate yourself using blankets to ensure the feet are pointing straight back towards the wall behind you.

KNEELING POSE, SUPPORTED IN FRONT – *Adho Mukha Virasana*

This pose, also known as "child pose", creates a sense of well-being and can be practiced throughout pregnancy, all the way up to the day of the birth.

STEPS

1. Start with the kneeling pose (*figure 1.13*).
2. Bring your big toes together and separate your knees. Let your heels open to either side, so that the feet are horizontal and at the same height on the left and right side (*figure 1.17*).
3. Roll your calf muscles from inside to outside and sit comfortably on your feet.
4. Bend forward so the torso fits between the thighs.
5. To exit the pose, lift your upper body by pressing your hands to the floor.

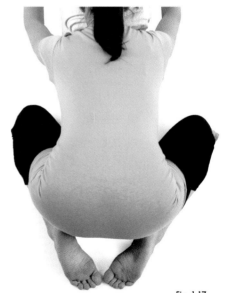

Fig. 1.17

Beneficial Effects:

- Rests your heart, helps to treat hypertension and diabetes.
- Allows breath to be felt everywhere in your torso: pelvic floor, lower back, spine, abdomen, and chest.
- Relieves your back and develops flexibility in the pelvis.

Caution or Special Support

According to your stage of pregnancy, adjust the height of the arm support, or rest your upper body on a chair (*figure 1.18*). For more comfort, place a blanket under your buttocks or over your heels (*figure 1.19*).

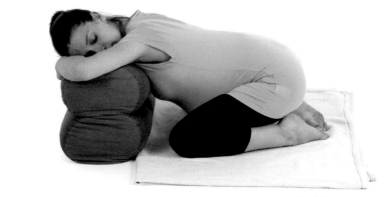

Fig. 1.18

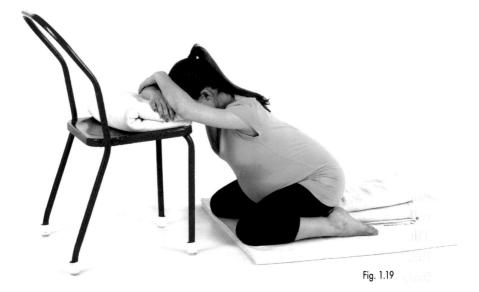

Fig. 1.19

TRUSTING BIRTH WITH THE BONAPACE METHOD

This pose is excellent for allowing your baby to descend into your pelvis at the moment of birth. The pressure that the baby's head puts on the cervix facilitates cervical dilation. Practicing this pose during pregnancy will help you develop strength and flexibility so that you can use this pose during the birth. As it is demanding, practice this with supports under the buttocks. Keep your balance by holding on to a scarf secured around your birth partner, a stair railing or the ledge of a window.

STEPS

1. Face the wall in the standing pose (*figure 1.2*). Place your feet a bit wider than your pelvis, and stand about 27 inches (70 cm) from the wall.
   - Feet flat on the floor, weight evenly distributed among the three points of your feet.
   - Lengthen your toes without tensing them.
   - Your feet are parallel and heels are in line with one another.
   - Stretch and lift your kneecaps by firming the quadriceps (thigh muscles).
   - Roll your thighs from the outside inwards to release the sacrum (the bone at the base of your spine).
   - Point the sacrum toward the floor. Keep the sacrum in a neutral position, not arched back or tucked under.
   - Lift your belly and gently tuck the lower ribs in.
   - Lengthen your spine and lift your chest.
   - Open your shoulders and chest by lifting the arms on either side of the body, palms to the sky.
   - Lower the shoulder blades, turn your palms and lower your arms so that they are alongside your body (*figure 1.2*).
   - Your head and neck are straight. Face and eyes are soft (*figure 1.3*).
2. If you have access to secure straps (or a window ledge, furniture, etc.), hold on to them and bend your legs while pushing your knees out sideways to let the abdomen through (*figure 1.20*).
3. Press your heels into the floor and the buttocks into the semi-rigid support.
4. Adjust the height of the support if your heels are lifting. Use a support, such as a rolled newspaper or magazine under the heels.
5. Tilt your body forward slightly.
6. Relax the head, shoulders and back.
7. Breathe normally.

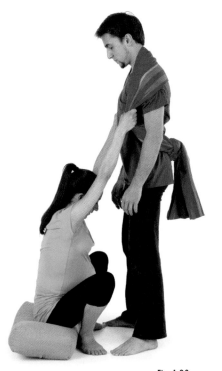

Fig. 1.20

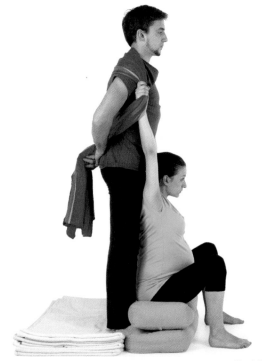

Fig. 1.21

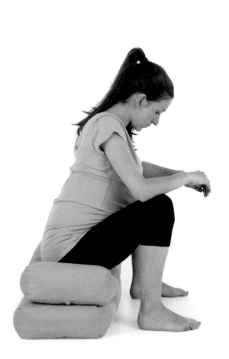

Fig. 1.22

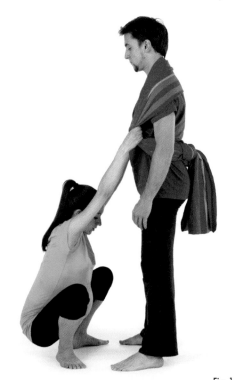

Fig. 1.23

TRUSTING BIRTH WITH THE BONAPACE METHOD

This pose can be practiced with the arms suspended above the body (*figure 1.21*) or placed against the knees (*figure 1.22*). As you increase the flexibility of your pelvis, you can reduce the height of the supports under your buttocks (*figure 1.23*).

Beneficial Effects:

- ◆ Promotes breathing when your arms are suspended.
- ◆ Promotes relaxation of the pelvis and back due to flexion (bending) of the legs.
- ◆ Promotes the baby's descent into the pelvis during labor.

> **PLEASE ENSURE THAT:**
> - Your back is lengthened.
> - Your legs are spread apart.
> - Your buttocks are relaxed.

Caution or Special Support

It is best not to practice this pose during the first trimester of pregnancy because the placenta is not yet well attached to the uterus. Avoid pushing in this pose until you enter the bearing down and birthing stage.

HORIZONTAL POSES

Whenever you are reclined on your back and you wish to get up, observe the following precautions. They will protect your back and your abs while preventing dizziness caused by abrupt position changes.

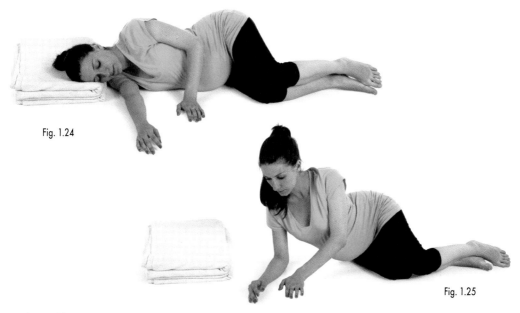

Fig. 1.24

Fig. 1.25

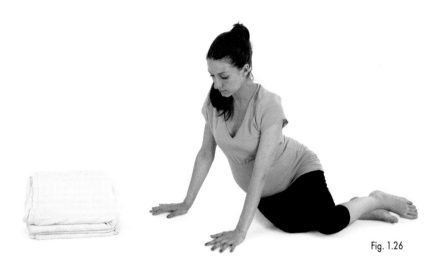

Fig. 1.26

STEPS

1. Lying on your back, bend your legs.
2. Turn your body to the side and roll your head without lifting it *(figure 1.24)*.
3. Support yourself with both hands on the floor and lift the body *(figure 1.25 and 1.26)*.

SUPINE POSE WITH LEGS UP A WALL - *Viparita Karani Mudra*

This is a complete pose with numerous benefits, proposed here for your relaxation. It can be practiced throughout pregnancy.

STEPS

1. Place your semi-rigid supports, or blankets stacked on top of each other against a wall. Your supports should be about 10 inches (25 cm) high. You can support your head and shoulders with a blanket.
2. Sit on your mat, with your left hip and left foot resting against the wall, next to your supports. Roll on your back. Place your feet on the wall.
3. Breathing and bringing the supports toward you, lift your buttocks and place them on the support.
4. Slide your buttocks closer to the wall. Your buttocks and the back of your pelvis rest entirely on the supports. Your shoulders are resting on the supports. Adjust the supports slightly closer to your waist if it feels uncomfortable.

5. Stretch your legs out by sliding the heels first. Despite the inversion, the buttocks and legs should be in a state of rest (*figure 1.27*).
6. Breathe and roll the shoulders back and toward the hips. Extend your arms out to either side of you.
7. Stay in this position for 5 minutes, gradually increasing the time to 10 minutes. Close your eyes and relax.
8. To come out of the pose, open your eyes, bend your knees, keeping your feet pressed against the wall (*figure 1.28*) and slide your buttocks to the floor (*figure 1.29*).
9. Roll onto your side. After a few seconds, come to a seated position by supporting yourself on your hands..

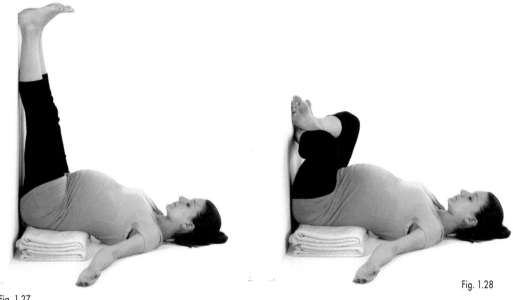

Fig. 1.28

Fig. 1.27

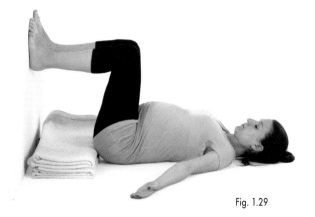

Fig. 1.29

Beneficial Effects:

◆ Calms and promotes quick relaxation and recuperation.

◆ Increases your appetite, which is positive if you have nausea or vomiting.

◆ Reduces edema in the legs.

Caution or Special Support

If this pose causes discomfort, nausea or a unpleasant sensation, stop the practice and replace with Shavasana (*figure 1.31*).

SUPINE POSE - *Viparita Karani Mudra*

This is a variation of the preceding pose, which is used for relaxation at the end of practice.

STEPS

1. Prepare the props needed for the position. Place a blanket where your head will be, a semi-rigid cushion beside you, and chairs side by side in front of you to support your legs. Lie on your back, rolling to the side, knees bent, with your hips close to the chairs.
2. Lift your legs one at a time and place one calf on each chair, resting the entire surface of the calves on the chairs (*figure 1.30*).
3. Exhale, raise your buttocks and while holding the ends of the bolster with your hands, place your buttocks on top. The buttocks are entirely supported. The pelvis, coccyx, and belly are parallel to the floor.
4. Place your blanket under your head so that the forehead is slightly sloping down toward the chest.

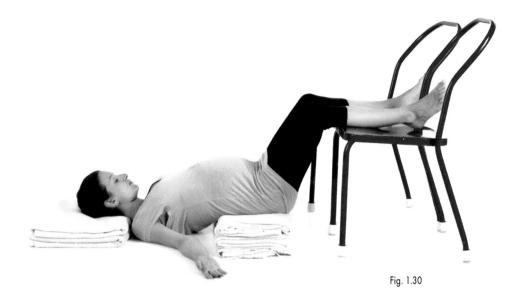

Fig. 1.30

5. To open the chest, roll the shoulders back and down toward the waist. Extend your arms to your sides and turn your palms facing the ceiling.
6. Close your eyes and relax for 5 to 10 minutes.
7. To exit the pose, open your eyes and lift your pelvis to remove the rigid cushion.
8. Bring your knees toward your chest, stretch the arms above the head and roll to the side.
9. After a few seconds, support yourself with your hands to bring yourself to a sitting position.

PLEASE ENSURE THAT:
- Your back is lengthened.
- Your buttocks rest on the support.
- Your chest is open and your shoulder blades are not protruding in the back.

Beneficial Effects:
- Calms and promotes quick relaxation and recuperation.
- Increases appetite, which is beneficial if you have nausea or vomiting.
- Reduces edema in the legs.

Relaxation poses are designed to relax the body and calm the mind. Enjoy this time to focus on your feelings, communicate with your baby and pay attention to your breath.

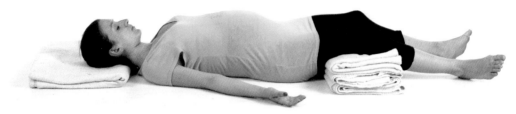

Fig. 1.31

STEPS

1. Place a semi-rigid support under the knees. Place a blanket under your head (the forehead is slightly sloping down toward the chest).
2. Lie on your back by placing your hands on the floor to one side and using your thighs to roll onto your side. Avoid using your rectus abdominis (large abdominal muscles) to roll onto your back.
3. Widen your buttocks by grabbing the flesh under your sit bones and gently stretching them to the sides so that your lower back is well-supported by the floor.
4. Release your legs and feet and allow them to fall outward. To open your chest, roll the shoulders back and down toward your waist.
5. Extend your arms to your sides and turn your palms facing the ceiling. Arms are at a 45 degree angle from the body.
6. Make sure the head is centered and in line with the spine.
7. Pay attention to the symmetry of your body. Allow your upper eyelids to lower onto the bottom ones, relax your eyes in their sockets and release all tension accumulated around the eyes, temples, and lips.
8. Use this time to rest.
9. To exit the pose, push the support under the knees with the feet and roll on the side. Use your hands to pull yourself up to a sitting position.

Beneficial Effects:

- Brings energy to your body and mind.
- Releases tensions.
- Facilitates contact with breathing and sensations.

Caution or Special Support
Variant of Supine Pose

If you feel discomfort while practicing the supine pose, it might be because of compression of the vena cava, the main vein along your back that ensures the return of blood from the pelvis to the heart. In that case, opt for the side-lying pose, which can be practiced up until the very end of pregnancy (*figure 1.32*).

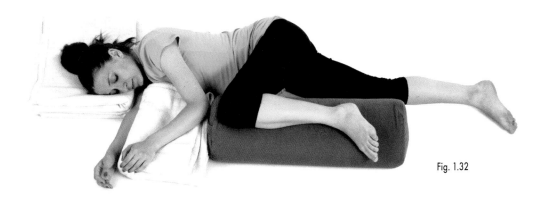

Fig. 1.32

PLEASE ENSURE THAT:
- One of your knees is at a 90 degree angle to the other leg.
- The bent leg is supported along its whole length.

ADDRESSING COMMON COMPLAINTS

In the following paragraphs, you will find solutions to some common problems that may occur during your pregnancy.

Magnesium Deficiency

Magnesium is a dietary element that is indispensable to life. It is responsible for numerous processes, including muscle function and blood clotting. It works together with calcium. Magnesium relaxes muscles, while calcium stimulates their contraction. Magnesium helps to build and repair body tissues. In optimal quantities, it can help to prevent hypertension[10], leg cramps[11] and hospitalisation during pregnancy[12].

A significant part of the population suffers from magnesium deficiency. Because only 1% of the body's magnesium is actually in the blood, this deficiency cannot be diagnosed with blood tests.

It is easier to detect a deficiency by the presence of certain symptoms. Constipation, leg cramps, spasms, fatigue, insomnia, muscular tension, back pain, neck or jaw pain, headaches, nausea, vomiting and loss of appetite can all be symptoms of magnesium deficiency.

The recommended daily dose of magnesium is from 300 to 450 mg for women between the ages of 19 and 40. However, when certain symptoms are present, it is sometimes necessary to double or triple your magnesium intake. Although a healthy diet may meet the body's magnesium needs, certain unhealthy or low-quality foods, and some medications, may make supplementation necessary. Almonds, cashews, pumpkin and sunflower seeds, spinach, salmon are all rich in magnesium. Consult a naturopath for advice.

Constipation

Constipation afflicts some pregnant women. If this is the case for you, add foods rich in fiber (whole wheat, corn bran, oat bran), as well as vegetables, fresh and dried fruit (prunes, figs, grapes, apricots, etc.) to your diet, and adjust your magnesium intake.

You can also promote the digestive process by practicing the squatting position (*figure 1.22*) and keeping physically active.

Calf Cramps

Calf cramps are frequent and painful. To prevent them, adjust your magnesium intake, avoid pointing your toes, and watch your circulation. To ease calf cramps, practice the standing pose (*figure 1.3*) and the seated pose with legs extended (*figure 1.9*). You can also stretch your calves as described below.

STEPS

1. Standing with one foot flat on the floor, slide the foot of the painful leg back as far as possible (*figure 1.33*).
2. Gently bend your other leg.
3. Come back to the starting position.
4. Repeat several times.

Find someone to support you in doing this stretch.

STEPS

1. Lying down, extend the painful leg.
2. Ask your partner to gently support your knee with one hand and use the other hand to put pressure on the sole of your foot, until it is at a 90 degree angle to your leg (*figure 1.34*).
3. Maintain this pressure for 5-10 seconds.
4. Repeat several times.

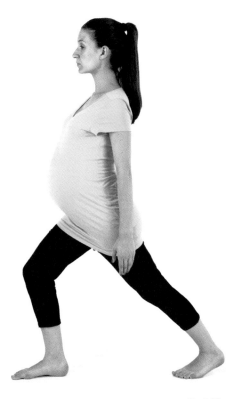

Fig. 1.33

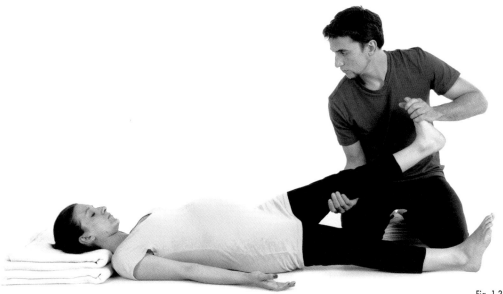

Fig. 1.34

BACK PAIN

In order to prevent back pain, here are some tips for protecting the abdominal muscles, facilitating relaxation, lifting heavy loads, and releasing tension in the lower body.

Protecting the Abdominal Muscles

The abdominal wall is made up of multiple layers of muscle. The surface layer is composed of the rectus abdominis. This is a set of muscles that, due to pregnancy or intense straining, tend to move away from the central line.

In order to prevent the displacement of the rectus abdominis and the descent of the organs:

◆ Practice yoga regularly.
◆ Avoid certain movements (*figures 1.35 and 1.36*).
◆ Roll onto your side when moving from a supine to seated position.

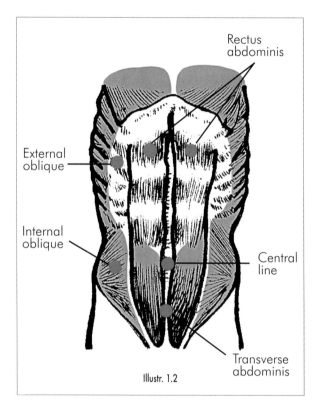

Illustr. 1.2

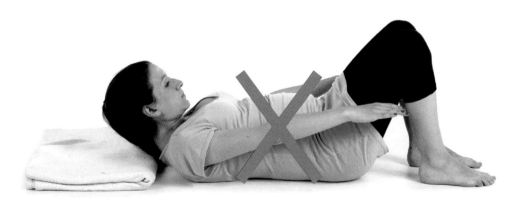

Fig. 1.35

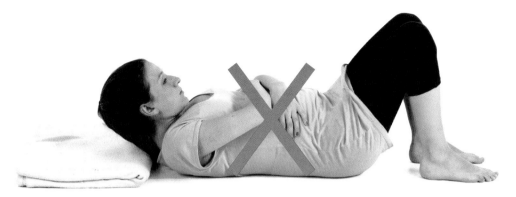

Fig. 1.36

- Before any exertion, contract the perineum (area between the vagina and rectum) on the exhalation by tensing your legs and buttocks.
- Lift only a reasonable amount of weight (maximum 22 lbs./10 kg).

Relaxing on the Floor or in Bed

To facilitate relaxing on the floor or in bed and to avoid the accumulation of tension in the back, practice this position.

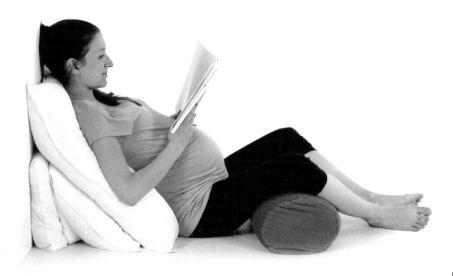

Fig. 1.37

STEPS

1. Fold a pillow in half and place it against the wall. It will provide lumbar (lower back) support.
2. Place another pillow vertically, to support your shoulders (*figure 1.37*).
3. Legs apart and bent, place two pillows under the knees, the first folded in half and the second placed straight.
4. Breathe softly and relax.

Appropriate Lifting

In order to prevent back pain and keep your balance, here are some tips that you can put into practice each time you lift something heavy[13].

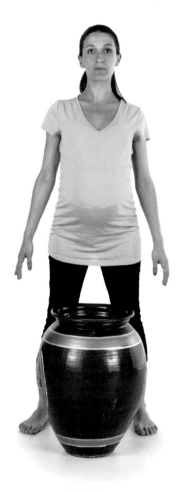

Fig. 1.38

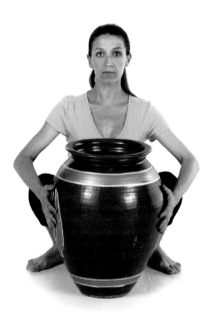

Fig. 1.39

TRUSTING BIRTH WITH THE BONAPACE METHOD

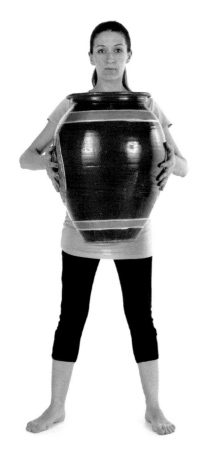

Fig. 1.40

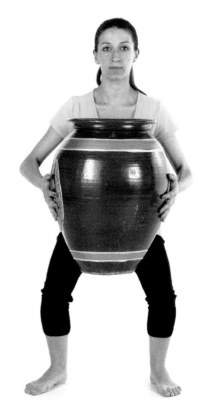

Fig. 1.41

1. Stand facing the object to be lifted, and bring your center of gravity close to the object (*figure 1.38*).
2. Spread feet and knees apart to increase balance and make room for the abdomen.
3. Point your toes in the direction you will be moving. Do not turn your body while lifting the object.
4. Bend your knees while keeping your back straight, and use the strength in your legs to lift the object (*figure 1.39*).
5. Make sure you have a solid grip on the object. Use the base of your fingers and the palms of your hands to make contact with the largest surface area possible.
6. Keep the arms outstretched. Use them to keep the object in balance, but not to lift it.
7. Flatten the pelvis (lengthen the back) and then lock it in this position, as in the standing pose (*figure 1.3*). This will distribute the weight over the entire spine.

8. Move your head back, chin pointing toward the chest. This movement helps to keep the back straight.
9. Lift the object on a deep and complete exhalation, after having first contracted the perineum[14,15] (*figures 1.40 and 1.41*).

Lifting a Young Child
STEPS

1. Hold the child against you (*figure 1.42*).
2. Bend your legs.
3. Keep your back straight.
4. Lower the sacrum as in the standing pose (*figure 1.2*).

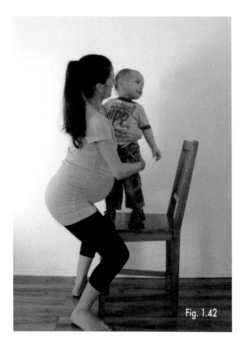

Fig. 1.42

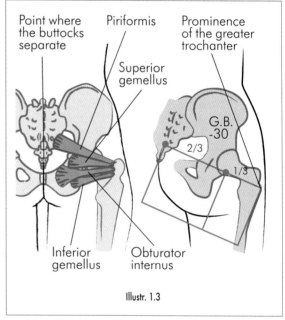

Illustr. 1.3

Painful Gluteal Muscles

The gluteal muscles (muscles of the buttocks) are the location of a large portion of lower-body tension. To relax them, we will make use of acupuncture point G.B.-30 (*illustration 1.3*) to disperse accumulated tension. The more sensitive the area is to touch, the more useful the massage will be.

Gluteal Muscle Massage

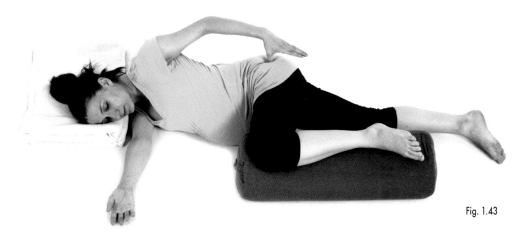

Fig. 1.43

STEPS
1. Lie down on your right side.
2. Extend your right leg on the floor.
3. Bend your left leg on top of the right.
4. Rest your left foot behind the right knee.
5. You can place a pillow under your left knee.

Finding point G.B.-30 (illustration 1.3)
STEPS
1. Move along the leg with your hand flat until you feel the greater trochanter protruding at the upper end of your femur (large bone in your leg). Place your finger just above this bump.
2. Imagine the point where the buttocks separate.
3. Imagine a line between these two points, and divide it into three equal parts.
4. The point that marks the first third, near the greater trochanter, is G.B.-30. Apply pressure with a finger for 30 seconds (*figure 1.43*).
5. Release.
6. Repeat three times.

If the stimulation is too uncomfortable, massage using the palm of your hand rather than your finger. Hands flat, make large movements starting at G.B.-30 and moving up toward the ribs (*figures 1.44 and 1.45*), and then down along the side of the leg (*figures 1.46 and 1.47*). Tension is thus spread over a larger surface area without creating any discomfort.

You can apply Chinese eucalyptus- or menthol-based oil, or red or white tiger balm, to relax these muscles.

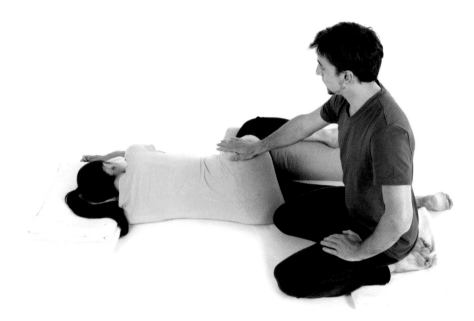

Fig. 1.44

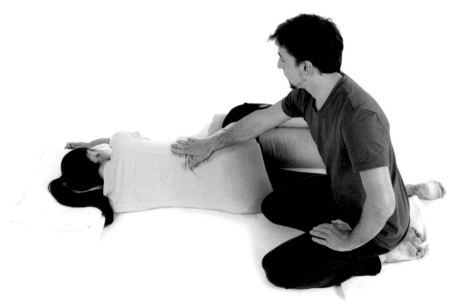

Fig. 1.45

TRUSTING BIRTH WITH THE BONAPACE METHOD

The more sensitive G.B.-30 is, the more useful it is to massage it frequently and deeply for a few minutes, every day if possible. G.B.-30 is extremely useful for relieving discomfort in the lower body during pregnancy, and for decreasing pain during labor rushes. See chapter 6, p. 141 to learn more.

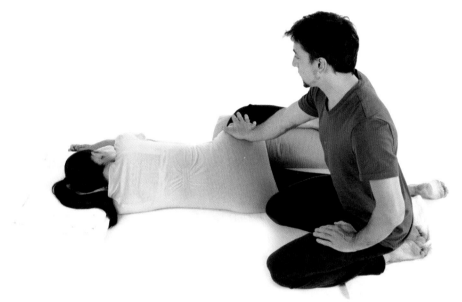

Fig. 1.46

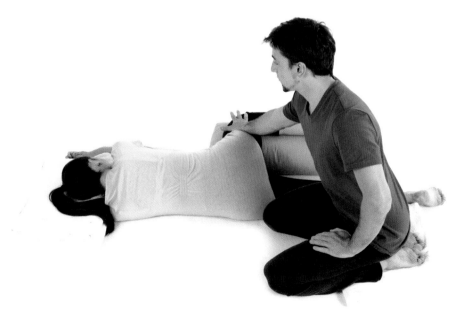

Fig. 1.47

A Tensed Perineum

The perineum is a series of complex muscles that close the pelvis. It is made up of the superficial perineum, which includes the sphincter muscles (vulva, urinary orifice, anus), and the deep perineum (*illustration 1.4*). The deep perineum is composed of extremely resistant muscles that work against the downward pressure of the internal organs. It acts as a trampoline and is particularly called upon during pregnancy and birth.

A tightened deep perineum increases pain during pregnancy and birth. The following exercise will help you to

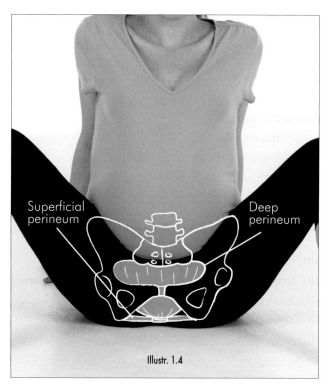

Superficial perineum

Deep perineum

Illustr. 1.4

become aware of the difference between a tensed and a relaxed deep perineum. During birth, relax your buttocks and your tongue. Exhale without resistance.

STEPS

1. Take a seated position, back straight (*illustration 1.4*).
2. Contract your buttocks on an exhalation. Observe the sensations in your belly, buttocks, sacrum, and finally perineum. This is the tightened deep perineum.
3. To release, let your tongue and your buttocks be soft. The belly is soft, the perineum is supple, and the sacrum can breathe.
4. If you find it difficult to sense the deep perineum, breathe (exhale) through the mouth with lips pursed. The pressure that you feel at the bottom of the pelvis corresponds to the contraction of the deep perineum, in reaction to the pressure caused by the breath[16].
5. To relax your perineum, practice the same breathing, but with relaxed lips. This time, relax the muscles of the buttocks. There is a less painful sensation in the perineum because you have relaxed it.

During pregnancy, create space in your sacrum by practicing the standing pose (*figure 1.2*). This pose prevents tension in the piriformis muscle and compression of the sciatic nerve. You should not feel any weight on the perineum except at the end of pregnancy, when the baby starts to descend into the pelvis, or during exertion (vomiting, sneezing, coughing). Consult your care provider if this is of concern and you need support.

Perineal Muscle Massage

This massage targets part of the superficial perineum and the lower part of the deep perineum that you can feel at the entrance of the vagina. It offers a way for you to prepare these muscles for the stretching that will be needed during the delivery of the baby. It also allows for minimizing the risk of tearing during the birth and of continued perineal pain during the postnatal period[17].

Another goal of the massage is to stretch the pelvic floor muscles and to desensitize them so that you can push without being disturbed by the burning sensation caused by the delivery. Finally, the massage allows the woman to get to know this part of the body that many women are not familiar with and do not feel comfortable touching.

In order to be effective, the massage should be practiced regularly, starting at the thirty-second week, or even earlier[18]. This massage can be done either by the woman or by her partner, whichever is most comfortable for both. It is important that the two of you are in agreement. During the massage, imagine that the muscles are releasing, and repeat to yourself silently: "I am opening the passage for my baby", "my perineum is supple and relaxed".

This 3-4 minute massage can be done in a hot bath, in the shower, or in bed. If you are having trouble finding the perineum and the opening of the vagina, find a comfortable position on some pillows, and, with the help of a mirror, examine the different parts of the vulva. The massage will be done on the region of the perineum between the opening of the vagina and the anus (*illustration 1.5*). To help you, use a sweet almond oil, coconut oil, oil with vitamin E, or a natural lubricant.

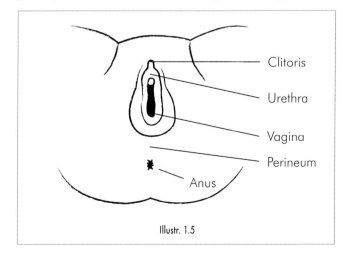

Illustr. 1.5

STEPS

1. Wash your hands.
2. Oil the perineum and the inner edge of the vagina.
3. Insert the index finger and the middle finger or the thumb into the vagina (1.2 to 1.6 inches/ 3 to 4 cm).
4. Make half-circles by pressing on the pelvic floor toward the anus and the sides for 30 seconds (*illustration 1.6*).
5. Delicately relax the opening by pressing and pulling with the help of the index finger and middle finger, until there is a light burning or prickling sensation (*illustration 1.7*).
6. Maintain this pressure and this stretching for 1 minute so that the zone becomes numb (becomes less sensitive). You will notice the effects after 2 or 3 weeks of massage.
7. Massage the perineum for 30 seconds by making circular or sweeping motions (*illustration 1.8*). If applicable, focus your movements on the scar of a previous episiotomy, since this tissue is less elastic (*illustration 1.9*).

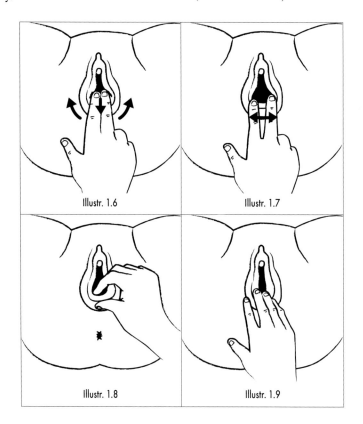

Illustr. 1.6

Illustr. 1.7

Illustr. 1.8

Illustr. 1.9

8. Relax the facial muscles, the mouth and the legs during the massage. Visualize the perineum stretching and repeat to yourself "I am opening the passage for my baby. My perineum is supple and relaxed."

9. Wash your hand and the vulva.

Caution or Special Support

Do not practice perineal massage if you have had herpes lesions or have suffered from active herpes during your current pregnancy, or if your waters have broken prematurely. Consult your care provider first.

THE BABY'S POSITION IN THE UTERUS

The optimal positioning of the baby at the beginning of labor is with the top of your baby's head facing downwards, and your baby's back facing the front of your belly (the occiput anterior position, illustration 1.10).

This optimal presentation allows your baby to incline its head by pulling in its chin and move through the various narrow passages of the pelvis with the smallest part of its head. With this positioning, labor starts better, is shorter, and less intense.

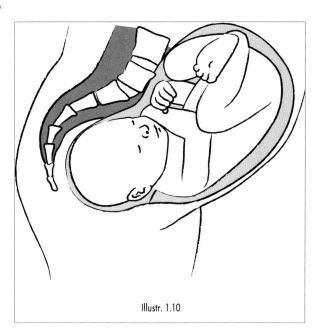

Illustr. 1.10

Some Tips for Promoting Optimal Positioning of the Baby

- Practice yoga poses daily, as this helps open the pelvis, creating the space necessary to receive the baby. When joints are flexible and the pelvis is symmetrical and on the proper axis, it is easier for the baby to engage in the optimal manner.
- Stay active and, most importantly, practice positions where the upper body is leaning forward, which will help rotate the baby's back (the heaviest part of its body) toward the front (*figure 1.48*).
- Avoid the sofa, or anything that makes you slouch. Sit on the floor instead, with your back lengthened (see the section on sitting postures, p. 21).

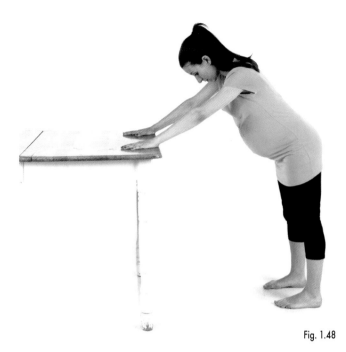

Fig. 1.48

- Avoid sleeping on your back as much as possible.
- Do not cross your legs, as this will force the pelvis out of equilibrium and change the axis.
- Once the baby is well-aligned in the axis of the pelvis, go for long walks to keep the baby in position.

Despite these precautions, it is possible that the baby presents in numerous variants of the occiput anterior position. The most common deviations are:

- The baby's back is facing your back (occiput posterior position).
- The baby's buttocks are facing downwards (breech position).

Practice the following movements which certain scientific studies have shown to be effective. At the same time, it would be wise to consult with your care provider (midwife, doctor, acupuncturist, osteopath, or obstetrician), who will have other positions or options to recommend to you.

A Baby in the Occiput Posterior Position

Sometimes your baby is positioned head-down with its back facing your back (*illustration 1.11*).

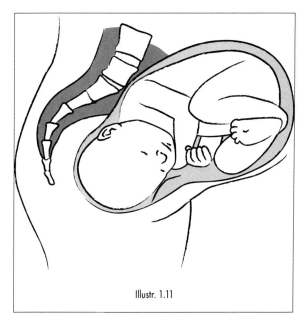

Illustr. 1.11

ON ALL FOURS

To help an occiput posterior baby turn his back toward your belly, get on all fours and let your belly hang down (*figure 1.49*). At the same time, practice light rocking motions of the pelvis[19].

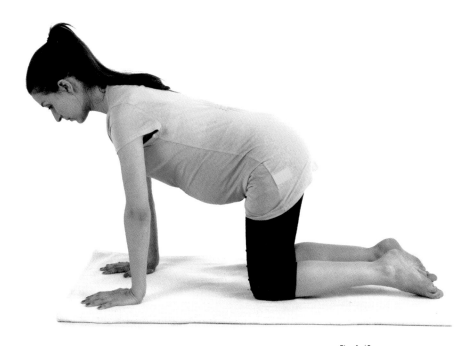

Fig. 1.49

A Breech Baby

By around 36 weeks, the baby is usually positioned head-down. If it isn't, practicing the following positions will frequently allow the baby's buttocks to disengage from your pelvis to facilitate the rotation of the head downwards. These postures are not advised for women who suffer from hypertension, and when the baby already has its head downward.

KNEELING POSE WITH HEAD TO THE FLOOR AND BUTTOCKS LIFTED

Multiple studies[20,21] have shown that when the kneeling pose with head to the floor and buttocks lifted is practiced three times a day for 15 minutes each, starting at the 36th or 37th week, the probability of turning a breech baby is greater than that of women who do not practice this position.

STEPS
1. Come to a kneeling position, keeping your shoulders close to the floor (*figure 1.50*).
2. Stay in this position for 2-5 minutes.

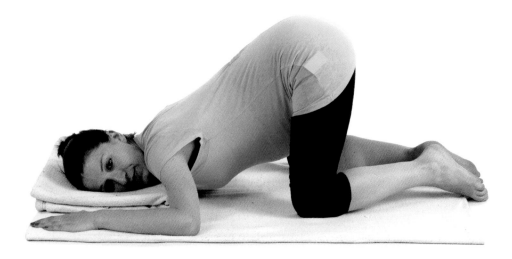

Fig. 1.50

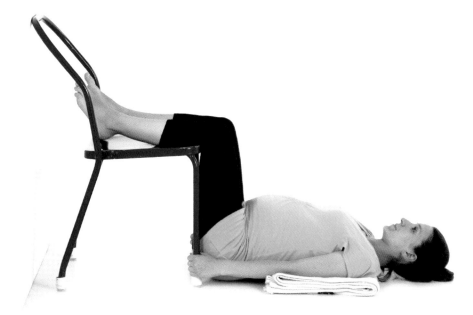

Fig. 1.51

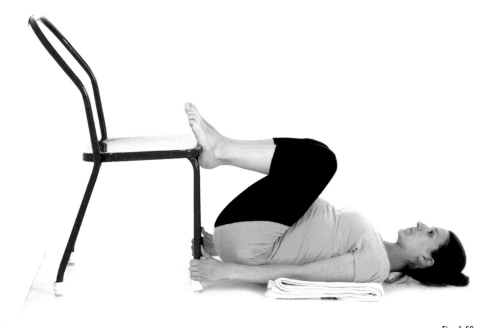

Fig. 1.52

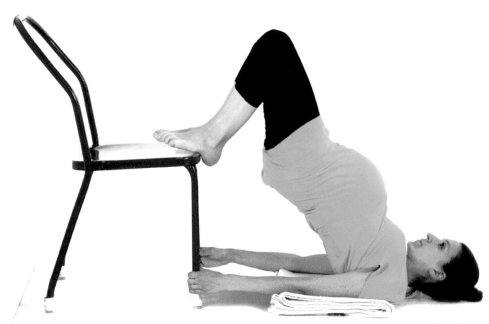

Fig. 1.53

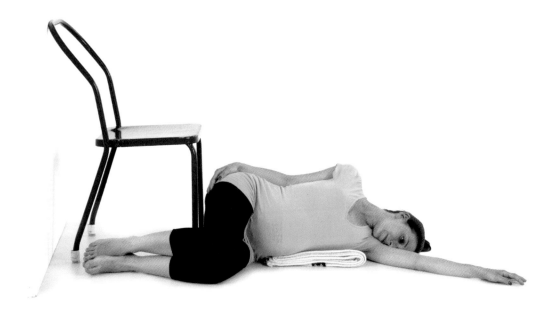

Fig. 1.54

TRUSTING BIRTH WITH THE BONAPACE METHOD

STEPS

1. Place the back of a chair against a wall.
2. Place one or more blankets where your shoulders will rest on the floor. In the final position, the shoulders should be supported by the blanket, relieving the pressure on the cervical vertebrae (neck) (*figure 1.51*).
3. Sit in front of the chair.
4. Place your ankles on the seat and bring your buttocks close to the chair.
5. Grasp the feet of the chair with your hands and stretch your arms. Lower your upper body onto the blanket (*figure 1.51*).
6. Place your feet on the edge of the chair (*figure 1.52*).
7. Adjust the distance of the blankets so that the back of your hairline (at the neck) touches the edge of the blankets. Roll onto your side and repeat the steps from the beginning if needed.
8. Breathe out and lift the pelvis (*figure 1.53*).
9. Roll your shoulders outwards to open the chest.
10. Keep this position for 10 to 15 seconds.
11. Slowly lower your pelvis to the floor, let go of the chair, lift your arms, and roll onto your side (*figure 1.54*).
12. Rest briefly on your side before coming to a seated position.

Results may appear in the three weeks following the beginning of your practice.

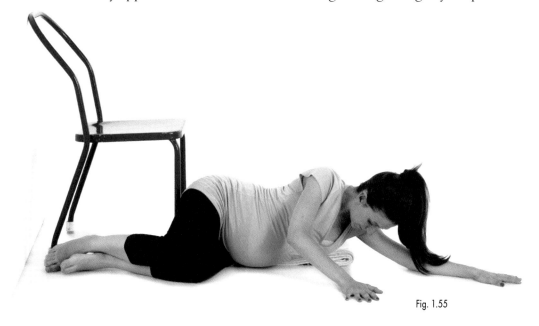

Fig. 1.55

PRACTICAL EXERCISES

Here is a 20-minute yoga routine that I recommend you do daily. Practiced regularly, these poses are beneficial: they improve your quality of life by relieving discomfort, and they contribute to reducing complications during pregnancy and birth.

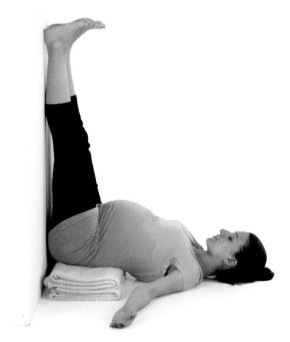

1. SUPINE POSE WITH LEGS UP A WALL
(Viparita Karani Mudra)
(see p.36)

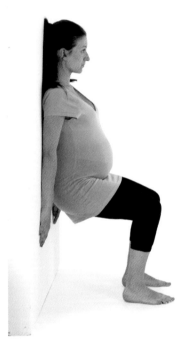

2. SEATED POSE SUPPORTED BY A WALL
(Utkatasana)
(see p.22)

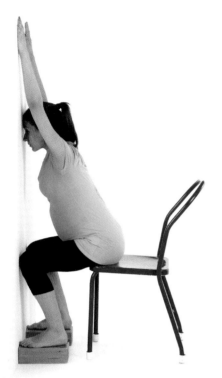

3. SEATED POSE ON A CHAIR, SUPPORTED BY A WALL
(see p.21)

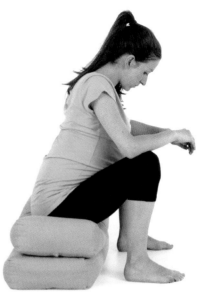

4. SQUATTING POSE
(Malasana)
(see p.33)

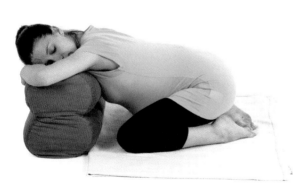

5. KNEELING POSE, SUPPORTED IN FRONT
(Adho Mukha Virasana)
(see p.31)

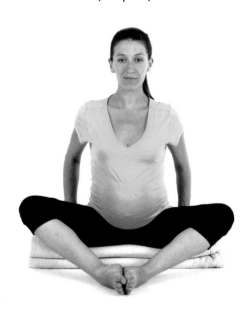

6. SEATED POSE WITH LEGS IN BUTTERFLY POSITION
(Badha Konasana)
(see p.26)

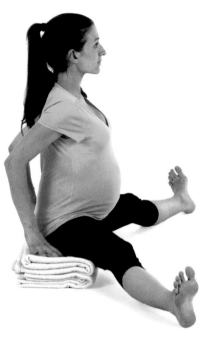

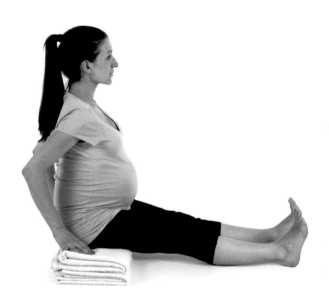

7. SEATED POSE, LEGS APART
(Upavishta Konasana)
(see p. 27)

8. SEATED POSE WITH LEGS STRAIGHT AHEAD
(Dandasana)
(see p.24)

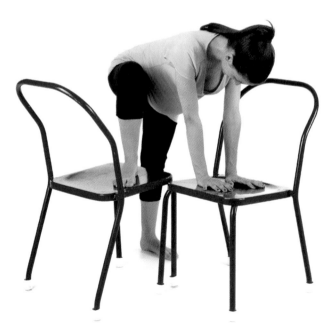

9. STANDING POSE WITH LEG TO THE SIDE
(Marychyasana 1)
(see p.19)

TRUSTING BIRTH WITH THE BONAPACE METHOD

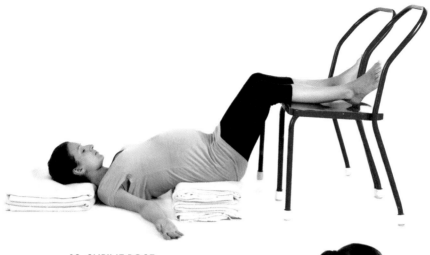

10. SUPINE POSE
(Viparita Karani Mudra)
(see p. 38)

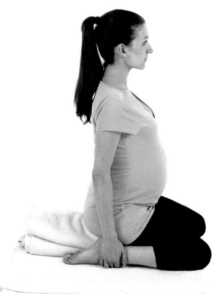

11. KNEELING POSE
(Virasana)
(see p. 29)

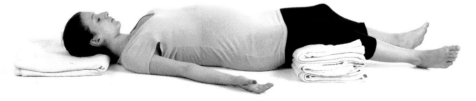

12. RELAXATION POSE
(Shavasana)
(see p. 40)

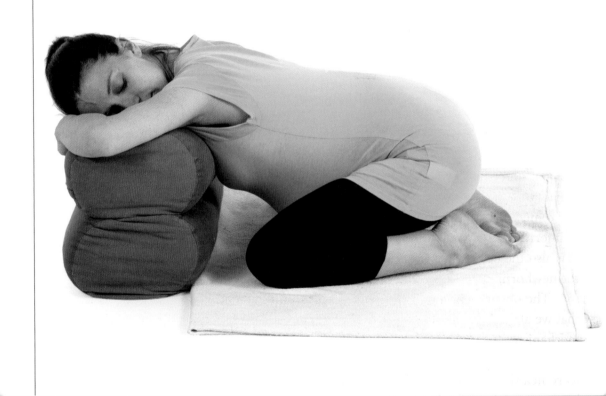

Chapter 2

PAIN MODULATION

Giving birth is an intense event. When you are expecting, everyone will tell you their experience, and the stories you hear are not always the most joyous. Some people call this the "hair salon syndrome". What I would like to emphasize is that your pregnancy and childbirth experience is unique to you. Your experience will be influenced by numerous physiological and psychological factors. To stay focused on your pregnancy, I encourage you to choose and filter the information to which you are exposed.

Often, we are worried about pain. Will we have the resources necessary to face it? Why suffer when there are pharmacological solutions that, most of the time, relieve 100% of the pain? It is true that the sensations of birth are intense[22]. However, they are not the sum total of the birth experience. It is an important moment that a woman will remember all her life, and it is an opportunity for self-discovery and the activation of internal mechanisms and resources that she may not have known she has access to. It is also the beginning of a relationship of love and attachment between parents and the newborn.

The phenomenon of pain is fascinating, but what is even more so is the capacity that we all have to modify these intense messages. The discovery of pain modulation mechanisms sheds light on the way in which women have dealt with pain for millennia.

In the last few decades, a birth was considered successful if the mother and baby were healthy and the birth was pain-free. However, when we begin to look at the longer-term view of a childbirth experience, starting with the postpartum period, then even further to ensure the survival of our species over time, it's important to address the larger issues at hand. Besides healthy mother and baby, it is also necessary to ensure the attachment between mother and baby and the establishment of successful breastfeeding. Both of these require much special care. Protecting the establishment of breastfeeding is critical, as it is sometimes the only option available to women to feed their child. We must therefore consider the potential impact of each act or intervention during the childbirth process on the following three poles: health, attachment, and breastfeeding. Non-pharmacological comfort measures are effective, safe, and free of undesirable side-effects. This is very important for women and their babies because they do not disturb the delicate balance between these three poles.

This chapter stands on four premises:

1. Giving birth is an intense experience.
2. Each woman has all the necessary internal mechanisms and resources to work with the intense sensations.
3. In order to effectively activate the sensation-modulating mechanisms, preparation and support are desirable. In fact, these mechanisms are frequently unknown or forgotten, and the modern context in which women give birth does not promote them.
4. It is possible that the mechanisms are not sufficient to reduce the intense sensations of rushes (contractions). In such cases, pharmacological approaches may help to reduce the intensity.

Summary of Chapter 2: Pain Modulation

OBJECTIVE	METHOD
Understand the role of intense sensations during labor and birth	◆ Understand the origin and the use of the intense sensations of birth ◆ Learn the components of pain
Become familiar with the mechanisms of pain modulation	◆ Learn recent discoveries in pain modulation
Understand why and how pain modulation techniques work: poses, breathing, massages, relaxation, mental imagery, environment, placebo, scents, music, support	◆ Learn various pain modulation techniques

Understanding the phenomenon of pain helps the woman and her partner to work with the intense sensations of rushes (contractions).

We will look into the internal mechanisms and resources that help you modulate (or alter) these sensations. But first, we will look at the factors that influence labor sensations, including the origin and usefulness of these sensations.

PAIN

It is worthwhile to examine your worries, fears, beliefs and values about pain. Recognizing that strong sensations serve a purpose, and that they play a role during birth, influences your perception and experience of this important event.

The Roles of Pain

Pain is defined as "an unpleasant sensory and emotional experience associated with actual or potential tissue damage, or described in terms of such damage"[23]. In general, pain plays a fundamental role in protecting us from real or potential dangers. It tells us that something important is happening and persuades us to seek help. It is at the origin of the majority of medical consultations.

Contrary to other types of pain, the strong sensations that a woman experiences in labor do not signify a threat, danger, illness or an anomaly. Rather, they let her know that an extraordinary event is in the making in her body, and encourage her to find a safe and peaceful place to give birth. They force her to stop what she is doing, to become aware of the importance of the impending event: the coming into existence of a human being.

Pain also provides important information about the progress of labor. When a woman is able to vocalize and change positions when she feels like it, her behavior can identify the progress of labor. When the mother feels an unpleasant pressure in her body, she will seek a different position. This adjustment is frequently useful in helping the baby move through the passages of the pelvis that lead to the outside world. Without the aid of pharmacology (or drugs), the fetus ejection reflex (a reflex that enables the baby to exit the birth canal without assistance) may manifest itself[24]. It is these distinct and intense sensations that the mother feels in the moment that guide her in her effort to push her baby out.

A woman who is able to respond to these intense signals effectively, by using her internal mechanisms and resources, feels a sense of great satisfaction. This reinforces her feeling of competence. It also strengthens her confidence in being able to meet the challenges of becoming a new parent[25].

In medicine, the negative cascade of obstetrical interventions that may occur when pain is not well-managed is sometimes documented. The cascade often unfurls as such: stress-fear, anxiety, pain, epidural or analgesics (pain relief drugs), synthetic hormones, reduction of sensations, forceps, vacuum extraction, episiotomy, etc. On the other hand, a positive cascade may occur when the woman and her partner prepare for and experience a birth in which they have the perception of having done their best. It could be described as follows: a mother and her partner who are prepared experience the labor together, work with the rushes by using multiple internal mechanisms, feel themselves to be 'actors' and not 'observers' of the birth, are proud of themselves and of each other, have an increased feeling of personal efficacy (self-esteem), which strengthens their partnership and their capacity to be good parents.

The Origin of Pain

Even though it's true that fear exacerbates the intense sensations of birth, it is important to clarify that other physiological factors unrelated to fear are at the origin of these sensations. During the first stage of labor, cervical dilation, the expansion of the lower part of the uterus and the pressure on adjacent structures activate the fibers responsible for potentially painful sensations[26]. Here, the trajectory followed by the nociceptive signal (signal that indicates potential pain) is typical of 'referred pain', which is to say a pain that manifests at the site where the pain originates and elsewhere.

The uterus, an organ, is relatively insensitive; significant stretching does not cause pain to it, but a referred pain, corresponding to the surfaces of the body linked to the nerve segments that enter the spinal cord at the same level as those of the uterus. Unable to distinguish the origin of the signals, the brain sends painful messages to all the surfaces corresponding to these nerve segments. This explains the intense sensations felt in the lower belly and lower back during a rush.

During the second stage of labor, the intense sensations are caused by pelvic traction, by the stretching of the perineal muscles and pelvic cavity muscles, and also by the strong pressure on the lower back's nerve roots. The perception of these sensations is transmitted through the pudendal nerve and is fast and localized, especially in the regions of the perineum and anus, the lower part of the sacrum, the thighs, and the lower legs.

As opposed to other types of pain, the pain linked to rushes doesn't usually indicate the presence of a pathology. This pain does not signify a deviation from a healthy, normal, or efficient condition. The force of the rush does not 'break' anything inside the body. It serves rather as a guide that helps the labor progress and acts with the body's other tools to help it adapt to this physiological process.

Factors that Influence Pain Perception

Fear and anxiety about birth are among the factors that have the strongest influence on the experience of pain. An accurate understanding of the mechanisms associated with the physiological processes of labor and birth reduces fear and anxiety, and therefore sensations. When the mother feels protected and safe, she lets go and abandons herself to the rushes, which facilitates labor.

TRUSTING BIRTH WITH THE BONAPACE METHOD

Also, the uninterrupted presence of a prepared partner near the woman contributes to reassuring and relieving her of fear or anxiety[27,28]. The more confident she is in her skills for dealing with birth, the better her reactions will be[29,30]. The mother experiences similar positive effects from the support of others including a doula[31] (professional birth companion), a close partner, friend, or family member, or of medical staff (doctors, midwives, nurses) who offer a wide variety of tools. Researchers have shown that continued physical, emotional and moral support contribute to improving the mother's satisfaction and the outcome of the birth[32]. The improvements include a reduction in the need for interventions including cesareans, use of forceps, vacuum extraction, pain medication, synthetic oxytocin (e.g. Pitocin), etc.

Prenatal preparation that includes physical, emotional and psychological preparation will play an important role decoding how your body perceives the sensations of labor.

Eliminate Pain, or Work with it?

In general, the health professionals who surround a woman in labor are well-meaning. Besides intervening in order to promote health and security for mother and child, they want to help relieve the woman's pain. Central to this medical model is the elimination of pain, operating on the assumption that pain is not useful and that the woman's satisfaction depends on its elimination. According to this model, if the baby and the mother are healthy and the woman did not experience pain, she must therefore be very satisfied with her birth. However, research shows that the woman's satisfaction with birth depends on four factors:

- her relationship with the care personnel;
- the quantity of support that she receives from them during labor and birth;
- her participation in decision-making;
- the taking into account of her personal expectations and her birth wishes[33].

If she wants to experiment with different options to work with her intense sensations (bath, massage, positions, breathing) and is not supported in this, she will in all likelihood be disappointed. Scientists propose replacing the "pain elimination" paradigm with the "working with pain" paradigm[34]. In all cases, it is not acceptable for the mother to suffer, since pain that is too intense and lasts too long can adversely affect the mother and her baby[35], as well as the progress of labor[36,37].

Suffering is the inability to activate one's own internal mechanisms for relieving pain, or an insufficient amount of resources for dealing with the situation[38]. Yielding to sensations, making loud noises, moving around and breathing strongly do not necessarily indicate maternal distress.

In order to prevent suffering, I suggest the use of Dr. Serge Marchand's circular model of pain as a tool to decode the intense sensations experienced by a woman in labor.

The Circular Model of Pain

The circular model of pain, created by Dr. Serge Marchand[39], illustrates the components of pain, and how they correlate to each other.

Pain is composed of at least four components:

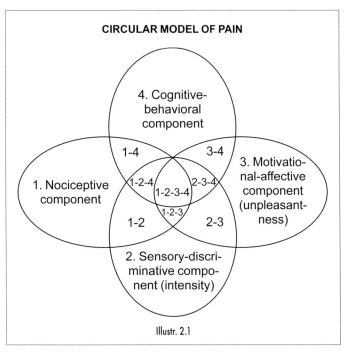

CIRCULAR MODEL OF PAIN

Illustr. 2.1

1. The **nociceptive component** is the real or potential injury. It is not always present, or known. In the case of birth, it consists of the stretching of the cervix, ligaments, muscles, structures and tissues, even if there are no real injuries per se.

2. The **sensory-discriminative (physical) component** allows for the feeling of the intensity and threshold of the pain. It can be modulated (or altered) by different processes, such as painful and painless massage, movement, baths and pharmaceutical means (e.g. epidural or drugs).

3. The **motivational-affective (psychological) component** allows for the judgment of the unpleasantness of the pain. Even if this component is related to the physiological component, it is much more easily modified by psychological techniques[40]. Distraction, support, emotions, relaxation, scents, self-hypnosis and thoughts, are all techniques that modulate (or alter) the unpleasant aspect of pain. It is thanks to this component that we can know whether the person "suffers" or is "working with" with her pain.

The intensity and unpleasantness of pain are components that are supported by two separate and distinct nervous pathways. Thus, the same pain can be perceived as being very painful but not very unpleasant, and vice versa. The pain associated with a joyous event, such as birth, is frequently more intense than it is unpleasant[41]. Women in labor who work well with these sensations will tell you that what they feel is very intense (component 2: intensity), but that they are doing well (component 3: unpleasantness). A woman who no longer feels her rushes due to an epidural, although she had planned to work with her pain, may be relieved of the intensity of her pain (component 2), while still experiencing an unpleasant emotional pain (component 3).

4. The **cognitive-behavioral component** is the way in which the person expresses their experience of pain. This component is strongly influenced by cultural factors. Family is, by far, the most important source of conditioning when it comes to dealing with pain. Memory of past painful experiences (e.g. our own, or those of our mother), socially acceptable emotional reactions to pain, our understanding of pain and methods for working with it are all conditioned by our cultural environment. If we are interested in understanding how a woman experiences her rushes, her behavior might be misleading since it is expressed via learned conditioning, influenced by her culture, her experience, and her environment. For example, Native American women do not express themselves much during labor, because in their culture it is believed that shouting or crying out chases away the spirit of the baby which would incarnate its physical body.

We must therefore avoid presuming and quantifying the sensations a woman feels, and rather ask her to evaluate them[42]. This can be done by inquiring how she is doing, if needed. Because it is a matter of perception, only the woman in labor can say whether she is doing well or not.

Therefore, the circular model of pain suggests two concepts:

1. The components are not necessarily all present when there is pain.
2. Each component can be addressed using different methods.

Sometimes **all four components of pain are present**, for example in the case of a wound (component 1) that causes intense (component 2) and unpleasant (component 3) pain that is expressed via crying (component 4). If this injury occurs during an important match in the Stanley Cup playoffs, when the player is absorbed in the fight, there might be an injury (1) that is neither intensely painful (2) nor unpleasant (3) and is not accompanied by behavior such as crying (4). At the end of the ordeal, when the player's attention is no longer absorbed by the game, the other components (2, 3, 4) will surface. When one loses a loved one, even though there is no injury (1), one feels a pain that is frequently intense and unpleasant and one expresses it via grimaces and crying (2, 3, 4). Before resorting to an epidural or pain altering drugs, measure the intensity (component 2) and unpleasantness (component 3) of the pain on a scale from 0 to 100. This will help you objectively evaluate what type of help you need. A high unpleasant component can show suffering and the need for support that increases the use of your internal mechanisms and resources to reduce pain, or the use of pharmacological pain-relieving drugs.

THREE NON-PHARMACOLOGICAL MECHANISMS THAT RELIEVE PAIN DURING LABOR AND BIRTH

For thousands of years, we have used numerous non-pharmacological techniques to relieve pain. Thanks to advances in scientific knowledge, it is now possible to explain how these different techniques work to reduce pain.

Here are the three non-pharmacological mechanisms that are capable of transforming the perception of pain[43]:

1. non-painful stimulation of the painful zone
2. painful stimulation of the painful zone
3. mental and thought control of the central nervous system

Scientific evaluations of non-pharmacological techniques show that they are safe and can relieve pain to different degrees[44]. Since the effectiveness varies from person to person, it is advisable to learn multiple techniques in order to have indispensable tools during pregnancy and birth.

Table 2.1 – The Three Non-Pharmacological Mechanisms for Pain Relief

THREE PRINCIPAL MECHANISMS	TECHNIQUE	ACTIVATION OF THE MECHANISM	EFFECTS ON THE COMPONENTS	DURATION OF THE EFFECT
• Non-painful stimulation of the painful zone • To be used between and during rushes	• Light massage • Bath or shower • Positions/movement • Ball • Hot or cold compress • Yoga poses	• Light massage of the painful zone will cause non-painful-fibers in the marrow to block some of the fibers that transmit pain messages	• Works solely on the zone that is stimulated • Mainly modulates (or alters) the intensity of pain	• Lasts mainly during the stimulation
• Painful stimulation of a location other than the painful zone • To be used during the entire duration of the rush	• Painful massage • Acupressure • Sterile water Injection • Acupuncture • Ice	• Painful stimulation triggers the secretion of endorphins, which drown the pain and only leave a painful sensation in the stimulated zone	• Works on all painful areas of the body except the stimulated area • Mainly modulates the intensity of pain	• Works during and after the stimulation
• Mental and thought control of the central nervous system • To be used between and during rushes	• Continued support • Structuring of thought • Breathing • Relaxation • Mental imagery • Believing in the technique (placebo) • Environment • Scents/aromatherapy • Music	• Pain is modulated by the structures of the brain that are responsible for memory and emotion.	• Works on all areas of the body • Mainly modulates the unpleasant component of pain	• Works mainly during and after practice

Non-painful Stimulation of the Painful Zone

Light massage of the painful zone will cause non-pain-fibers in the marrow to block some of the fibers that transmit pain messages[45]. This reduces the overwhelming perception of intense pain at this site. It also introduces the perception of a non-painful sensation to the same site. Light stimulation of the painful zone can be done by light massage, a jet of air (blowing on the painful area), pleasant warm water (taking a bath or shower), heat or cold (applying a 'magic bag') or movement (moving around).

Light Massage

A light massage of the painful zone transforms the perception of the sensations in this area. It is used mainly between rushes, and, if needed, during them.

Bath or Shower

A bath is considered the epidural of Quebec midwives. It allows the woman to relax, to float, to move freely and to reduce the stress hormones that inhibit rushes[46,47]. Bathing is a safe technique, both for the mother and for the baby[48]. It can be used during the dilation phase (first stage) and during the delivery (second stage). The temperature of the water should be the same as that of the mother's body, and as much as possible, the belly should be submerged. Portable birthing pools can be rented for this purpose.

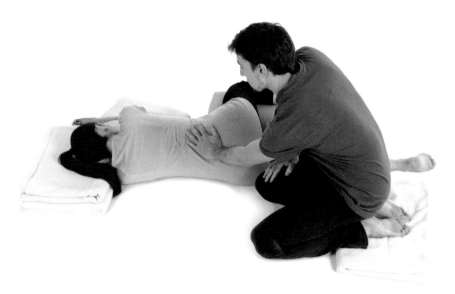

Fig. 2.1

Warm or Cool Compresses

Warm or cool compresses placed on the painful zone block part of the intense messages that are transmitted to the brain. They are used during and between rushes.

Yoga and Movement

Practicing different poses during labor (see chapters 1 and 5) reduces intense sensations, augments the effectiveness of rushes, and facilitates the descent of the baby into the pelvis, which makes labor easier and shorter[49,50,51,52]. The poses recommended in chapter 1 prepare the woman's body for birth, and those in chapter 5 help her to use movement to relieve discomfort.

Painful Stimulation of an Area Other than the Painful Zone

In ancient Greece, electric rays (sting rays) were used to relieve different types of pain[53,54], including pain from gout, rheumatism, and headaches. The barb was placed on the painful region and the electrical discharge that the patient received produced an immediate relief that lasted past the stimulation.

The principle of this technique is to create a painful stimulation at a site that may be distant from the original painful zone by activating certain neurons and inhibiting others simultaneously[55,56]. Today, we can use deep massage, acupuncture, injections, and other methods to introduce a secondary painful stimulation. When our body experiences this new pain, endorphins (an internally-produced morphine) are released. Pain from all sites in the body is inhibited by the endorphins, except for the pain that was introduced by this secondary painful stimulation. The endorphins produce a pain relief that lasts longer than the painful stimulation. This mechanism has no side effects, and even relieves pains that are resistant to conventional analgesics. This technique modulates (or alters) pain mainly by decreasing the intensity.

The techniques primarily used to activate this mechanism are acupressure (painful massage), acupuncture, the use of ice, and local injection of sterile water.

Acupressure

Acupressure is a deep (painful) massage of the acupuncture reflex zones[57,58]. This approach combines two mechanisms to facilitate labor: the benefits of Chinese medicine (pain relief and promotion of efficient labor) and the release of endorphins due to the creation of a second pain source.

During the entire rush, an intense deep massage stimulates certain acupuncture reflex points of the lower back, buttocks, feet, hands, and legs of the laboring woman (chapter 6).

Acupuncture

Acupuncture uses needles to stimulate precise points on the body in order to relieve pain. In labor, the needle stimulation introduces a second pain source and is sometimes inserted in a region of the body distant from the original source of labor-related pain. This brief stimulation can produce relief that lasts well beyond the period of insertion[59].

Ice

Applying ice is an easy way to create a second painful stimulation in any part of the body during a rush. It is only necessary that the sensation caused by the ice be strong.

Sterile Water Injection

The local injection of very small quantities of sterile water at the base of the back is an excellent way to reduce the intensity of pain[60]. This injection creates slight bulges right below the skin surface.

Sterile water must be injected by a care provider *during a rush* to create the second pain. Two injections provide relief for 90 to 120 minutes and act on all of the body's pains.

The injections are repeated as soon as the endorphins' effect wears off. This technique is used after having tried the other non-pharmacological approaches, since there is an intense and unpleasant feeling for a few seconds during the injection.

With this second mechanism, the second intense stimulation is always done during the rushes.

Mental and Thought Control of the Central Nervous System

Mental concentration techniques allow for the modulation (or altering) of pain messages and the inhibition of physiological and psychological reactions.

Controlling the nervous system transforms the perception of pain; it plays a dominant role in the management of pain. The transformation of the painful perception gives rise to the following phenomena:

- a modification of the message (sent from the pain point to the brain)
- the release of endorphins (from the brain to the body)

In the higher centers of the brain, pain messages establish direct and indirect links to other regions of the brain that are associated with memory and emotions. Therefore, images and messages that are found in those other regions influence the way in which the unpleasant aspect of pain will be perceived.

Techniques that make use of this mechanism rely mainly on physical and emotional support, structuring of thought, placebo, yoga, breathing, relaxation, mental imagery, scents and aromatherapy, the environment, and music.

Physical and Emotional Support

On its own, physical and emotional support has been shown to be one of the most important tools in reducing the need for pain medication and obstetrical interventions (e.g. cesarean deliveries, forceps, vacuum extraction, augmentation of labor, etc)[61]. This support must be continuous and be provided by a loving person who knows what to do and who works well with his or her own stress.

This mechanism is fundamental for helping the woman to create and stay in her zen state, a space (or "bubble") that allows her to experience her sensations calmly and confidently. This zen state or behavior is probably central to the reduction of all obstetrical interventions and the improvement of the mother's satisfaction with her birth experience.

Structuring of Thought

Structuring of thought consists of correctly reframing what exactly a woman believes birth implies. If, for the woman, a rush is synonymous with fear and anxiety, her sensations will feel very unpleasant. If, on the other hand, she sees rushes as both essential and positive, and if she is convinced that endogenous (internal) mechanisms are at work releasing morphine to relieve her, and that she has everything that is necessary to give birth safely, the unpleasant nature of the sensations will be greatly diminished.

Placebo

The role of placebo in the treatment of pain is becoming better known. A placebo is defined as the therapeutic effect obtained by the administration of a treatment that is not a treatment. Thus, only one condition is necessary for the placebo to work: that the patient and the person administering it believe that it will work.

The attitude and values of the care personnel with you during your labor constitute a powerful placebo. The more the care providers believe that non-pharmacological comfort measures are effective, and most importantly, believe that it is important for the parents to be satisfied during the postnatal period, the greater your confidence will be during labor. To ensure that this approach is effective, the pregnant woman should ask beforehand that she not be continuously offered pharmacological approaches to dealing with her labor, that rather her care providers wait until she requests them. She should choose care providers who believe in the numerous positive effects of non-pharmacological techniques during pregnancy and birth.

Yoga, Breathing, Relaxation and Mental Imagery

Yoga is an effective and comprehensive approach to well-being[62,63]. Through diligent practice of poses (chapter 1), conscious breathing (chapter 4), and relaxation (chapter 7), yoga develops one's capacity to concentrate and to relax.

Breathing works on different levels: first, to oxygenate and relax the tissues, and then, to divert attention. Certain studies show that women who know how to relax perceive less pain and need less intervention (e.g. forceps, vacuum extraction, etc.) to birth their babies[64].

Because it allows us to become aware of our reactions to pain and to modify them as needed, mental imagery (chapter 8) is a precious tool for preparing psychologically for birth. It helps to create realistic goals and to develop means to attain them, which contributes to making the birth a satisfying experience.

Scents and Aromatherapy

Although research has concluded that aromatherapy (the use of aromas derived from plants and flowers for therapeutic use) does not reduce pain during birth, researchers have shown that any perceived pleasant scent reduces pain much more than neutral or unpleasant odors[65]. This may be one of the reasons for the difference in perception between women who give birth at home, and those who give birth in a hospital. If the woman does not like the smell of her environment, and associates it with something negative (e.g. illness or injury), her mood will be affected, as will her pain perception.

To counter this phenomenon, the pregnant woman chooses a scent that she likes (e.g. the scent of lavender) and adds a couple of drops of the scent to a cloth. Each time she practices relaxation, she places the cloth near her face, so that she develops a positive association between the scent of lavender and the state of relaxation. During labor, she puts the same scent onto her clothing or a cloth, which, by association, improves her mood and reduces painful sensations.

A Safe Environment

Chapter 3 describes the way in which a cocktail of hormones is produced by the woman in labor. These hormones are released when she feels safe, that her intimacy is protected, and that she is not disturbed. Helping the woman to create her zen zone, with lowered lights, calm, warmth and intimacy, favors the release of hormones which make labor safe and easy.

Music

Although no study has shown music to have an important effect on diminishing intense sensations, if it pleases the pregnant woman and allows her to relax and divert her attention, it can certainly be useful to her. What is important is to choose music that she likes.

A recent study compared standard care approaches to non-pharmacological techniques grouped into the three mechanisms (i.e non-painful stimulation of the painful zone; painful stimulation of the painful zone; and mental and thought control of the central nervous system). It was found that when physical and emotional support are combined with at least one other mechanism, the frequency of obstetrical interventions (e.g. cesarean, forceps, vacuum extractions, epidural, synthetic oxytocin/Pitocin, etc) is reduced and maternal satisfaction is increased[66]. Regular practice of non-pharmacological comfort measures and belief in their effectiveness are ways to contribute to their success. If you wish to put these multiple techniques into practice, the pregnant woman should ask those surrounding her to support her in this project. She should invite them to prepare themselves with her, to have confidence in her, and to encourage her during labor and birth.

THE BONAPACE METHOD AND COMFORT MEASURES

The Bonapace method calls upon many techniques that, according to one study, reduce the intensity and unpleasantness of pain by nearly 45%, for both first-time mothers and those who have given birth before[67]. This research compares conventional birth preparation techniques with the Bonapace method. The active presence of the partner to support the mother is also an important part of this model.

Comfort measures have been around for millennia. Due to their effectiveness and innocuousness (i.e. absence of side effects), they are important tools that will allow you to fully experience your birth.

PRACTICAL EXERCISE: DAILY PAIN MODULATION

Be mindful of painful situations you experience in your daily life and practice the three pain modulation mechanisms (i.e non-painful stimulation of the painful zone; painful stimulation of the painful zone; and mental and thought control of the central nervous system). When a painful event occurs (e.g. visit to the dentist or esthetician), lightly massage the painful zone, if possible. Create a second pain during the first, and imagine something pleasant while relaxing your jaw and buttocks. Exhale deeply.

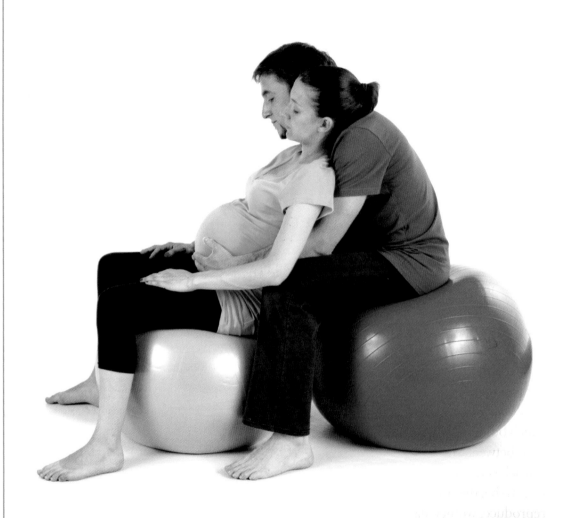

Chapter 3

THE BIRTH

Giving birth is a momentous event, to which a woman's body is adapted. For the majority of women, pregnancy and birth happen simply and safely. For others who need more care, the knowledge and tools of modern medicine are useful. Since women have been giving birth for millions of years, perpetuating our species, we can take for granted that nature planned everything so that reproduction happens successfully and safely.

In the previous chapter, you read that it is possible to modify potentially painful signals. You also learned that your body possesses strong mechanisms that diminish intense sensations and aid childbirth. In this chapter, you will see that nature has also provided another powerful system to help you: a delicate hormonal cocktail.

When the mother feels she is safe and protected, the hormones that she produces allow her and her baby to experience the birth safely and physiologically, which is to say in a manner that respects the innate functions of the body. These hormones are beneficial for both mother and baby. They contribute to creating an environment in which both mother and baby are healthy, and breastfeeding and attachment are established between the two. It is not enough that the mother and baby survive. Attachment is crucial, since the newborn needs lots of care. Breastfeeding has also been, and continues to be, the sole way for some women to feed their baby. For humans to continue to reproduce, women had to find pleasure not only in copulation, but also in giving birth.

Birth is a unique event of astounding simplicity and complexity that is not reflected in numbers or statistics. Although there are general rules that govern labor, each birth is unique, requiring us to adapt and welcome it with its particular variations. Knowing that your path may differ from the norm, pay attention to that which you can control (e.g. your attitude and your ability to live through the intense sensations) rather than worry about the components that you cannot control (e.g. the frequency and the intensity of rushes, cervical dilation, the baby's descent, etc.).

In this chapter, you will see that your body has many internal mechanisms and resources to facilitate labor. You will find all the information you need to recognize the beginning of active labor and the different stages it comprises. You will also learn the role of hormones and the conditions that maximize their effect. Most importantly, you will discover the ways in which you can create the most optimal environment for a safe, satisfying and pleasurable birth.

Summary of Chapter 3: The Birth

OBJECTIVE	METHOD
Create conditions that are favorable to the optimal process of labor	◆ Prepare mentally via knowledge of certain physiological and psychological aspects of birth ◆ Know the role that hormones play in an easy, satisfying and safe birth ◆ Create a physical and emotional environment that supports hormonal secretion (the woman feels undisturbed, safe and protected)
Promote continuous support of the woman in labor	◆ Prepare and establish a support team that meets the woman's need and is in agreement with her values
Make informed choices in regards to pain relief	◆ Know the effects of the epidural on the process of labor and birth, as well as effects on mother and baby
Participate actively in her own birth	◆ Make informed choices about birth location and care provider who will follow the pregnancy
Experience a satisfying birth	◆ Prepare a list of 'birth wishes' as a communication tool for all participants

As it relates to the birth, the woman's role is to:

1. Maintain confidence in her ability to give birth in a safe, easy and pleasant manner.
2. Create conditions that are favorable to the physiological process of her birth (i.e. preparing herself both physically and mentally, preparing her support team, practicing comfort measures, choosing her care providers, and choosing her place of birth).

3. Maximize the release of hormones by creating a zen zone (i.e. a "bubble") around herself.
4. Understand the process of labor and birth and know how to let go (i.e. to let nature take over).
5. Adopt a positive and confident attitude toward the different stages of labor.
6. Stay calm and concentrate on relaxation of the body by practicing conscious breathing and mental imagery.

The role of the companion consists of:

- Ensuring emotional and psychological support to the mother (e.g. being attentive, compassionate and loving).
- Providing her with physical support (e.g. giving light or intense massages, helping her establish helpful postures, and offering her all other comfort measures – as appropriate).
- Protecting the woman's zen state.
- Managing his or her own stress, and meeting his or her own needs, while supporting the mother.

THE PROCESS OF LABOR

The first chapter underlined the importance of strengthening, relaxing and relieving your body in order to prepare yourself to bring your baby into the world. In the weeks leading up to the birth, practice your yoga poses more frequently. In your free time, practice poses that promote optimal positioning of the baby in your pelvis (i.e. poses where your upper body is leaning forward, and positions where you are lying down on your side).

Pre-labor

Pre-labor[68] (also known as false labor) is a process that occurs at the end of pregnancy. This helps the woman to prepare for the intense sensations that she will experience during labor. The uterus hardens and stays contracted for a few minutes, at irregular intervals. It does not yield to pressure from the fingertips. These sensations are similar to menstrual cramps and the tension is located in the lower abdomen and the groin.

For certain women, these rushes will slowly transform the uterus, while for others it will take many hours of intense rushes to obtain this result. What is important is to accept and welcome the way in which your baby and your body are working together to help labor progress. In fact, you could see the pre-labor as a practice shot in golf. Not useless at all, this shot is important, even professionals use it to warm up, test their sensations and prepare themselves.

Table 3.1 presents the characteristics that distinguish pre-labor from labor.

Table 3.1 – Pre-labor and Labor

CHARACTERISTICS	PRE-LABOR	LABOR
Intervals between two rushes	◆ Irregular	◆ Regular ◆ Progressively shorter
Intensity of rushes	◆ Variable	◆ Progressively stronger
Effect of rest on rushes	◆ Sometimes stops them	◆ No stopping
Discharge	◆ Usually absent ◆ Sometimes loss of baby gel or mucus plug	◆ Usually present ◆ Light discharge with blood filaments (the cervix is effacing and dilating) ◆ Loss of baby gel or mucus plug, but not always ◆ Rupture of membranes
Cervix	◆ Sometimes no change	◆ Effacing ◆ Dilating

It is important not to confuse pre-labor with signs of premature labor (before week 36). Premature labor is characterized by more than four rushes per hour combined with pain or pressure in the lower abdomen and the groin.

Rushes

Real rushes are similar to preliminary rushes, but differ from them in their intensity and regularity. They present as a strong pressure of the lower stomach and groin, and diffuse at the lower back. Thanks to these, the cervix transforms. They come in waves, reaching a peak, then subsiding. They are rhythmic and continual.

When labor is well underway, rushes last about one minute, and stop for one minute. The *duration* is calculated from the beginning of the rush to the end of it. The *interval* is calculated from the beginning of one rush to the beginning of the next.

During the 10 to 15 seconds at the beginning and end of each rush, the intensity is lower, with the rush reaching its peak and staying there for 30 seconds. To help you stay in touch with your sensations, allow yourself to be carried by the wave. Avoid thoughts that produce discouragement such as calculations, forecasts, and expectations. Focus your thoughts on your baby or divert your attention by mentally counting your breaths, breathing out fully, and chanting the sound HU (pronounced HUE). This chant is done on the exhale, while relaxing the jaw and buttocks. Relax yourself and stay in the present moment. As soon as the wave is over, you will have a period of calm. Make the most of the break by resting and recharging your energy.

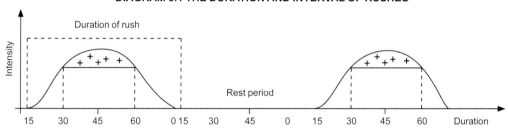

DIAGRAM 3.1 THE DURATION AND INTERVAL OF RUSHES

The Release of Hormones: A Mechanism Designed to Facilitate Birth

Fear, like thoughts, can upset the delicate balance of hormones. When a woman gave birth in the bush and perceived a danger or an important stressor, such as the aggressive approach of a wild animal, labor stopped in order to let her flee, and restarted once she felt safe again. The same thing happens today, except that the stressors are different. Giving birth in a strange place, with strangers, without one's own clothes and familiar landmarks can cause stress that is perceived as a menace. This perception of a threat can stop rushes until a woman resumes a feeling of security. This might be the reason why some women stop experiencing rushes when they arrive at the hospital.

To counter this effect, you should bring a few familiar objects from home (e.g. cushions, clothing, food, scents, balls, comfort objects). You can also arrange the room so that it promotes your intimacy and your zen state. Your birth partner can filter visitors and act as the guardian of your zen zone.

Besides being mechanisms that reduce pain, hormones are a powerful system that allows you to birth your baby with ease and safety. In fact, the hormones of love and pleasure (oxytocin), of transcendence and euphoria (beta-endorphins), of excitement (adrenaline and noradrenaline) and of mothering (prolactin)[69] work together during pregnancy and birth to create a delicate hormonal cocktail. A better understanding of this cocktail will help you to enter and stay in your zen state at the moment of birth.

An initial approach to activating these hormones is to create a birth environment that resembles the one in which you make love. It is the same hormones, the same body parts, the same sounds and same need for security and intimacy that are at play when making love, as they are when giving birth. For this reason, some researchers argue that the environment should also be similar[70]. We promote the secretion of hormones by creating a birth environment that is comfortable, warm, bathed in dimmed light, and where the woman's need for security and intimacy are respected.

A second method is to let the thinking part of your brain rest, and allow your focus to go to your sensations. In yoga, it is said that the mind is a liar. If a laboring woman starts calculating the minutes, the hours, or the centimeters of dilation, and concentrates on the fetal monitor, on what others are saying or thinking around her, she can easily leave her zen state. She can become afraid or worried and lose contact with what is real. To eliminate the frame of reference to time or progress, the calculating centers should be less active and the primal —or intuitive— brain more. All of these cortical stimulations force you out of your zen state. Imagine yourself in the middle of making love. You are swimming in oxytocin and beta-endorphins when suddenly your partner asks you for your mother's stew recipe. Have you lost the vibe? Not surprising. That is the effect of thoughts on hormones.

When a woman simply observes or is witnessing her sensations, allows herself to be carried by them, thinks about her baby, the birth, her "space of well-being", and repeats to herself that she is safe and that everything is well, she succeeds in letting go. The sensations appear and disappear. This is the reason why it is best to speak as little as possible, to avoid rational thoughts, and to cover the clock and the electrical monitors (if there are any) in order to avoid calculating.

Dr. Sarah Buckley[71] describes from a scientific and anthropological perspective the role of four hormones released by the mother and communicated to the baby via blood during the period of pregnancy and birth. Together, oxytocin, endorphins, catecholamines and prolactin make up the hormonal cocktail that ensures the security of both mother and child, promotes attachment and facilitates breastfeeding. It is the recipe that nature created to assure the survival of our species. These hormones are optimized when the mother feels safe, protected, and that her need for intimacy is respected.

Table 3.2 – The Role of the Main Hormones of Labor and Birth

HORMONE	ROLE
Oxytocin: the hormone of love, attachment, and well-being	**Psychological effects:** • Binds humans to each other by promoting love, attachment and well-being • Diminishes pain and softens memories related to pain • Is stimulated by 'skin to skin' contact (between mother and baby, and between mother And partner), visual contact with a loved one, touch, and stimulation of the nipples[72] **Physiological effects:** • Provokes rushes that dilate the cervix during labor • Protects the baby by diminishing the activity of nerve cells and the need for oxygen[73] • Contributes to the fetus ejection reflex[74,75] • Provokes rushes that reduce bleeding immediately after the birth[76] **Effects of medical interventions on oxytocin:** • Oxytocin levels drop when the mother does not feel safe, and when she is afraid • Oxytocin levels drop significantly in the presence of medical substances; this explains the frequent need to intensify labor with synthetic oxytocin (Syntocinon, Pitocin) after the administration of an epidural, for example • Oxytocin loses its psychological effects when it is replaced by a synthetic version (because the synthetic version is injected and does not cross the blood/brain barrier).

Beta-endor-phins: the hormones of pleasure, transcendence and relief	**Psychological effects:**
	• Modify the mother's state of consciousness by transporting her to 'another world'
	• Pass into the mother's milk, creating pleasure and a codependency[77] between mother and baby during nursing
	Physiological effects:
	• Reduce pain
	• Promote the release of prolactin (the hormone that prepares the breasts for nursing) during labor[78]
	Effects of medical interventions on beta-endorphins:
	• Beta-endorphins are greatly diminished by the administration of an epidural or analgesics[78a], and this diminution could have the following effects:
	  * Reduction of baby's relief during labor and immediately after the birth
	  * Reduction in the secretion of prolactin[78b] (maternal milk hormone) as well as the effects of codependence and pleasure transmitted by breastfeeding[78c].
	  * Medical substances can diminish the baby's ability to latch on and suckle, which delays the beginning of breastfeeding[79]

Catecholamins: hormones of stress and excitement	**Psychological effects:** • Augment the mother's level of attention and energy at the end of labor, giving her the strength to push **Physiological effects:** • Promote the fetus ejection reflex at the end of labor[80] • Protect the baby against a drop in oxygen during the pushing stage and prepare it to live in the physical world (catecholamins improve the baby's respiratory function, the regulation of essential components of the organism, and heat production)[81] **Effects of medical interventions on catecholamins:** • They may increase catecholamins during early labor, which will slow down or stop rushes[82]

Table 3.2 – The Role of the Main Hormones of Labor and Birth

HORMONE	ROLE
Prolactin	**Psychological effects:** • Promotes maternal behavior (vigilance and submission) in the woman so that she adapts to her role as mother[83] • Increases maternal tolerance to monotony • Is present in a father who takes care of his children **Physiological effects:** • Contributes to the production of maternal milk **Effects of medical interventions on prolactin:** • The secretion of prolactin could be diminished due to the decrease in beta-endorphins

THE UNFOLDING OF LABOR

"The process of birth starts with the cervix moving from back to front, softening, effacing and dilating. The baby's head turns and bends, and the baby descends and passes through the mother's pelvis to emerge into the open air[84]."

The labor of a woman giving birth is divided into at least three stages[85] (table 3.3).

Table 3.3 The Stages of Labor and Birth

1st stage	• Dilation of cervix from 1 to 10 cm • Comprised of two phases: latent phase and active phase
2nd stage	• Birth of the baby
3rd stage	• Birth of the placenta

First Stage of Labor: Cervical Dilation from 1 to 10 cm

During the first stage, physiological labor is divided into two phases: latent phase and active phase.

The Latent Phase

The latent phase is characterized by the slow and minimal dilation of the cervix and a slight descent of the baby. The frequency of rushes is irregular and the intensity may become considerable. Before dilating completely, the cervix thins under the effect of numerous rushes. This may take many hours.

During this period, be calm, and most importantly, patient. Stay at home, where you will be more comfortable. Eat, drink, and urinate as needed[86]. Continue your activities without overdoing it. It is completely normal that the cervix not dilate during this period, even after many hours of rushes. Make the best of moments of intimacy with your partner to prepare for the start of labor. Ina May Gaskin[87], an American midwife who has been practicing since the 1970s, recommends women do 'skin to skin' with their partners, since this closeness promotes the release of hormones that facilitate labor[88].

If the rushes intensify, breathe deeply. Exhaling empties the lungs (which prevents hyperventilation), raises the diaphragm (which reduces the pressure of the diaphragm on the uterus) and diverts attention (which reduces sensations). Chant the sound HU (pronounced HUE) (chapter 4) to help you exhale.

During stronger rushes, choose a comfortable position, relax the pelvis by rocking or swaying it if possible, and relax the deep perineum by releasing the buttocks.

The Partner's Role During the Latent Phase

During the rush, support the woman in her breathing practice (chapter 4) and create an intense stimulation in a reflex zone (chapter 6). Spend time with your partner. If she plans to give birth at home, check on the final preparations. If she is going to give birth at a birthing center or hospital, be sure to have prepared everything that you will need for your partner's comfort and your own (see Appendix 1: Birth Travel Bags and Baby Supplies Checklist)

The Active Phase

The cervix is now ripe, which is to say ready to open sufficiently to pass behind the baby's head. It is the effect of the rushes and the pressing of the baby's head that allows for the opening. Compared to the latent phase, the cervix dilates much more rapidly. The rushes will probably be longer and closer together.
At the beginning of active labor, the woman might:

- Have a sudden renewal of energy
- Feel strong sensations in her lower back and hips
- Have vaginal secretions
- Lose her baby gel (or 'mucus plug')
- Notice her membranes releasing (or 'water breaking')
- Notice a change in the duration and intensity of rushes
- Notice that resting has no slowing or stopping effect on rushes

Looking closer at these signs, we see that[89]:

- Some women feel a sudden renewal of energy that may be caused by a decrease in the level of progesterone produced by the placenta. To prevent becoming exhausted in labor, if this occurs, do not use up too much of this newfound energy.
- Lumbar (lower back) and sacroiliac (sacrum and pelvic) tensions may occur. These tensions become more intense due to the effect of relaxin, a hormone that softens the pelvic bone joints.
- Vaginal secretions may increase due to the effect of vaginal mucus congestion. Some women lose small amounts of blood. Caution: know the difference between normal blood loss and hemorrhaging. If you continuously lose small quantities of blood, communicate with your care provider and avoid exerting yourself.
- The baby gel or mucus plug is a gelatinous mass that resembles coagulated egg white. It blocks the opening of the cervix during pregnancy and protects the baby from vaginal microbes.
- The membranes (i.e amniotic sac) that envelop the baby may release, causing a colorless liquid to discharge from the vagina. This is amniotic fluid. Wear a sanitary pad to absorb the liquid. Lie down and let the liquid flow. Then, communicate with your care provider.
- Rushes change. They become more regular, more intense, and closer together as labor progresses. For the cervix to dilate completely, multiple intense rushes are needed (*illustrations 3.1 to 3.4*).

Turn your attention away from the clock, the monitors (if there are any) and technology, to avoid activating your cortex, the thinking part of your brain. Observe and witness your sensations. Have confidence in your hormones and in your capacity to use pain modulation techniques effectively. Your labor will take the time that it needs. Even if the sensations are very strong and you sometimes feel like something inside of you is breaking, nothing is. Women have evolved with mechanisms to birth safely. The sensations of birth are different than those of an illness or injury. These sensations are there to support the process. Be confident. TRUST! You, like all women, have what it takes to bring your baby into the world.

Remember that the strong sensations are useful for teaching you how to move and position yourself. Be proactive in finding what relieves you, one rush at a time. Intense doesn't necessarily mean bad. In your moments of distress, think about your baby who is benefiting from the beta-endorphins, the natural analgesics that are relieving and protecting your baby. Remember that it is the rushes that are causing the cervix

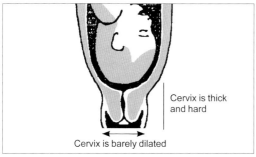

Cervix is thick and hard

Cervix is barely dilated

Illustr. 3.1

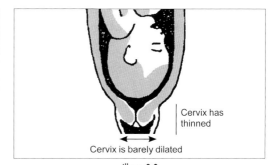

Cervix has thinned

Cervix is barely dilated

Illustr. 3.2

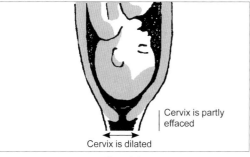

Cervix is partly effaced

Cervix is dilated

Illustr. 3.3

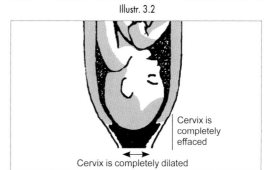

Cervix is completely effaced

Cervix is completely dilated

Illustr. 3.4

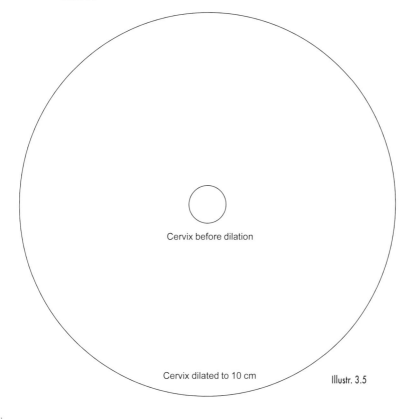

Cervix before dilation

Cervix dilated to 10 cm

Illustr. 3.5

to open, your baby to pass through the passageways, and you to give birth. Be zen! See illustration 3.5 for an example of a cervix dilated to 1 cm and 10 cm.

If you are planning to give birth somewhere other than at home, it is recommended to leave home when the pattern of rushes is 5-1-1: the rushes have occurred every *5 minutes* for *1 hour,* each one lasts *1 minute,* and they are intense enough that they demand all of your attention[90]. In case of doubt, call the hospital or your care provider.

WHEN TO LEAVE FOR THE HOSPITAL OR BIRTHING CENTER

If it is your first baby, arrive at the hospital or birthing center, or call:

1. When your rushes are regular, every five minutes for at least one hour, last about a minute, and each prevents you from talking and demands all your attention.
2. Or if you are leaking fluid (your waters have broken).

If it is your second or subsequent baby, take into account the duration of your first labor and discuss with your care provider. In principle, arrive at the hospital or birthing center when the rushes are regular, every 10 minutes for 1 hour, or if the membranes have ruptured or if you have bloody discharge.

During the rush, exhale deeply or chant the sound HU (pronounced HUE). Breathing allows you to concentrate on your sensations and divert your attention. Stay calm and rest between each rush. Relax the whole body, especially the abdomen, the legs and the buttocks. Ask your partner to shake your thighs and your buttocks if they are tense. This allows the perineum to relax so that it does not reflexively resist the pressure of rushes, which amplifies the intensity of the sensation.

Focus your attention on something other than the rush. Think about your baby. Create a second pain in a reflex zone (chapter 6). Try different positions to relieve discomfort with suspensions, supports, or by lying on your side or coming to a sitting or squatting position (chapter 5).

Remember that emotions are sometimes responsible for a long labor that does not progress.

"Ina May Gaskin[91] described the birth of a young woman for whom dilation was taking a long time. She asked the woman if something was bothering her. The young woman replied that when she married her partner, he refused to say the part of the vows that referred to being together for life. This made the woman feel insecure. Would the father still want to be with her after the birth of the baby? Unconsciously, she was holding back the baby to avoid facing this possibility. Ina May discussed the situation with the father and proposed celebrating a new ceremony on the spot. Once the vows were made, the young woman's cervix opened completely to allow the child to be born."

To help you use the energy of your emotions, I suggest the Emotional Freedom Technique (EFT) further on in this book (chapter 8).

The Partner's Role During the Active Phase

The role of the birth partner is of utmost importance during this phase. Due to the strength of her rushes, the woman's state of consciousness is frequently altered, which is beneficial for the mother and the baby. This is the effect of endorphins. When she is in her zen state, avoid disturbing her with questions. Witness the process and be prepared to offer comfort measures. Tune in to her needs.

1. Remind her that she has everything she needs to give birth.
2. Show her that you have confidence in her by saying "you're amazing and glowing; you're doing it; I trust you; I am in awe".
3. Reassure her. Protect her. Be her guardian. Watch over her.
4. Be loving and encourage her gently. Be understanding.
5. Create an atmosphere of calm and serenity.
6. Manage your own stress and anxiety.
7. Help her to practice breathing. Encourage her to concentrate on exhaling completely. Chant HU (pronounced HUE) with her.
8. During the rush, practice massages by creating a pain at a site other than the original painful area.
9. Between rushes, caress her body and give her affection.
10. As needed, lubricate her lips with oil.
11. Wipe her face with a sponge or cloth.
12. Work with her to find a comfortable position.
13. Suggest a bath.

14. Remember to relax, to stay calm and eat enough. Your support is essential to her.

Studies on continuous support by the father, a birth companion (doula), a member of the family or a care provider show that physical, moral and emotional support diminish the need for all obstetrical interventions and improve maternal health and satisfaction, as well as infant health[92]. This support helps the woman to stay in her bubble or zen state.

Solutions for Discomfort During the Active Phase

During the active phase, you may notice some unpleasant symptoms.

Nausea and vomiting: Women frequently prefer drinking liquids over eating. Taken at room temperature in small mouthfuls, water provides necessary hydration during labor. At the end of this book you will find a recipe for magnesium-rich broth (see Appendix 2: Recipes).

Irrational thoughts: Irrational thoughts are very useful, especially when they happen at the end of labor. They are activated by stress hormones and have the effect of galvanizing you to action to get the baby out. Work with these emotions and use them to activate your internal mechanisms. Continue to have confidence in yourself and stay focused on your breath. Follow your instinct. To help you to experience your intense emotions, practice the Emotional Freedom Technique (chapter 8).

Intense sweating and uncontrollable shivering: these sensations sometimes follow each other and create discomfort. Adjust your clothing accordingly. Exhale deeply and stay calm.

Chattering teeth and shaking legs: do leg-balancing movements. Lightly brush the inner thighs. Continue to practice breathing.

Second Stage of Labor: The Birth of the Baby

Increased levels of adrenaline and noradrenaline, the hormones of excitement and stress, play an important role at the end of labor. The stimulatory effect of these hormones increases the mother's energy, strength and vigilance and creates several powerful and involuntary rushes that birth the baby quickly and easily. This has been termed the fetus ejection reflex[93,94]. Observations suggest that this reflex may not be active when labor is disturbed. The fetus ejection reflex is augmented by intense rushes at the end of labor causing the baby to progress through the mother's pelvis (without the need to push). The stretching of tissues caused by the pressure of the baby's presenting part (i.e head or buttocks) activates specialized nerve fibers in the mother's lower vagina and cervix. These nerve fibers send a message to the brain, which releases a large quantity of oxytocin. The oxytocin creates more strong rushes which make the baby progress even further, causing additional stimulation of specialized nerve fibers. This feed-forward loop, known as the Ferguson reflex[95,96], is responsible for the elevated level of oxytocin released during the post-partum period and allows the mother to expel her baby easily. However, when medical substances are present, oxytocin levels see an important drop. This explains why this reflex is often absent in hospital maternity wards.

The fetus ejection reflex may be accompanied by other typical signs of increased stress hormones: increased muscular strength, dry mouth, an urgent need to stand up, and sometimes even intense verbal and non-verbal expressions. "Physiological fear" as described by Michel Odent[97] can manifest by expressions such as "I am dying; I am transcending!" In animals, elevated levels of catecholamines during this period causes a newborn protection mechanism which accentuates aggressive-defensive behavior in the female[98].

This fetus ejection reflex can be inhibited when one asks the mother to begin pushing before the reflex appears, or when the mother is disturbed by examinations, interventions, or cortical (the thinking part of the brain) stimulation when someone talks to her, by the proximity of strangers, and by medical substances, including synthetic oxytocin and the epidural.

In order to facilitate the fetus ejection reflex and the Ferguson reflex, create an intimate environment in which you feel you are in a zen zone – your "bubble". Listen to your sensations and wait for the baby to descend into the vagina before pushing. If the reflex starts, you do not have to do anything besides follow the irresistible urge to push. If the reflex does not occur, adopt a position that makes gravity work in your favor. Avoid lying on your back (chapter 5).

Third Stage of Labor: Delivering the Placenta

The delivery of the placenta usually occurs within the hour following the baby's birth. It usually requires little effort on the part of the mother. However, the birth is not complete until the placenta is delivered. To facilitate the expulsion of the placenta, maintain a calm environment, continue to protect your zen state, and avoid talking or using reason. Continue to practice techniques for modulating (or altering) intense sensations. Wait at least five minutes before cutting the baby's umbilical cord, or, better yet, wait for the placenta to be born. It is scientifically recognized that a third of the baby's blood stays in the placenta if the umbilical cord is clamped immediately after birth. In the minute following the birth, 50% of the blood is transfused, and in the first three minutes, the percentage increases to 90%[99]. Delaying cord clamping allows optimal blood transfer from the placenta to the baby, as well as a gentle respiratory transition for the baby. Being connected to the supply of placental blood even after the birth provides a secondary source of oxygen for the baby, and allows the baby time to adjust to using its lungs to breathe in the new environment outside of the womb.

EFFECTS OF THE EPIDURAL

Obstetrical interventions will influence your physiological hormonal cocktail to varying degrees. Let us look more precisely at the impact of the epidural on the mother and her baby, as well as concrete methods to reduce undesirable effects.

The epidural is the most effective and widely used pharmacological intervention in the West. It acts to reduce or eliminate pain by injecting medical substances near the nerves that transmit pain and are situated in the spinal cord. These substances reduce the nerve impulse of sensitive fibers, and, to a certain degree, the motor fibers that transmit messages to the muscles.

Although it is considered safe, more and more research tends to show that the epidural can have harmful effects. Disruption of the delicate hormonal balance, in particular the effect of the epidural on natural oxytocin, highlights an aspect of these effects.

A recent systematic review by the Cochrane Collaboration[100] attributes the following effects to the use of the epidural:

- An increased need for synthetic oxytocin;
- A prolonged second stage of labor;
- An increase in the rate of forceps and vacuum extraction use;
- And an increase in cesarean births due to fetal distress.

With the epidural, the fibers that are at the origin of the ejection reflex are numbed, which inhibits the feedback loop and the reflex itself. A woman under epidural must therefore use her own strength to birth the baby[101]. What is more, not feeling the pressure from the baby, which tells her how to move, and not being able to move freely (because of a decrease in sensations) does not help her get into a vertical position which would let gravity work in her favor. These different factors explain the prolongation of the second stage of labor and the higher likelihood of forceps and vacuum extraction use. The number of episiotomies (cutting of the perineal muscle) and lacerations is also increased[102].

There are only a few quality studies that document the impact of the epidural on breastfeeding. However, the majority of care providers would say they could generally recognize babies born to a mother who was under epidural by the baby's slow adaptation to breastfeeding. The placental barrier does not keep out medical substances administered to the mother while she is under epidural. These substances reach the baby, who has a harder time eliminating them than the mother, because of the immaturity of the baby's system[103]. His suckling reflexes and capacities are diminished, which makes breastfeeding more difficult[104].

Since the mother no longer feels pain under the epidural, her secretion of beta-endorphins, the analgesics that alter her state of consciousness[105] and produce prolactin, diminish greatly. Research shows that in the postpartum period, the level of endorphins is greatly diminished, if an epidural is administered. And, as we know, endorphins transmitted by the mother's milk give pleasure to both mother and baby, and create a relation of codependence between them.

After the intervention occurs, the hormonal cocktail is modified, the woman moves around less, and is confined to the IV (intravenous) drip. She is frequently attached to a fetal monitor and has her arterial blood pressure measured, which can affect her feeling of intimacy, because she feels observed.

To understand the impact of other obstetrical interventions on your hormonal cocktail, I invite you to consult these well-researched texts written by perinatal specialists[106,107,108].

Minimizing Undesirable Effects of the Epidural

Women's bodies are equipped with powerful mechanisms for dealing with the pain of labor rushes. Support, relaxation, painful and light massages, baths, and all other tools described in this book have proven effective. Don't forget that birth is full of surprises. You may feel intense sensations without an instant change in the cervix, and then suddenly the cervix dilates and opens quickly.

It is also possible that labor may be long and intense, which might cause the release of stress hormones (catecholamines) which prevent cervical dilation. In this case, an epidural can be an important ally, allowing the woman to relax and the cervix to dilate.

If, after having tried all comfort measures, an epidural is still needed, here are some suggestions for minimizing the undesirable side effects of this intervention:

1. Wait until labor is well underway before considering an epidural (some authors recommend waiting until cervical dilation is more than 4 cm). This way, you and your baby will benefit from the effect of hormones for at least part of the labor.

2. Do not aim for a 100% reduction in sensations. It is better to retain some sensation after receiving the epidural. Opt for low doses of medical substances. The lower the dose, the less it will affect your baby and your ability to establish breastfeeding.

3. Keep moving. Change positions, and avoid lying on your back. Your mobility will probably be limited, but move anyway by lying on one side and then the other, going on all fours, and kneeling.

4. Stay in your zen state with your partner or those who are accompanying you. Maintain contact with your baby.

5. Wait before pushing. Start pushing only when the baby's head has descended into the vagina[109].

6. Establish skin-to-skin contact with your baby starting at birth, to stimulate the release of natural oxytocin.

Identifying Your Needs and Making Choices

The goal of this book is to give you the tools and knowledge that will enable you to experience the birth of your baby as satisfying, pleasurable, and safe. From the start of your pregnancy, you will have an important decision to make: choosing the care providers who will accompany you for the duration of your pregnancy. Due to different realities in different regions and countries, you may not always have a choice. Your confidence in the care providers whose care you are in contributes to a normal birth.

A recent systematic review of scientific literature evaluated the impact of birth location on obstetric interventions. It first looked at non-standard birthing environments including: a maternity ward birthing room where the technological devices are camouflaged; a birthing unit outside of – but adjacent to – the maternity ward; and (more recently) it looked at rooms furnished and decorated to reduce cortical (i.e. thinking brain) stimulation and designed to maintain calm, freedom of movement, and intimacy. The non-standard birthing environments were compared to conventional hospital rooms where the bed is at the center, surrounded by technology. These are the results:

- A reduction in medical interventions
- A higher likelihood of spontaneous vaginal birth

- Greater satisfaction on the part of the mother
- Greater likelihood that the mother will continue to breastfeed in the first and second months following the birth
- No additional risk for either mother or child

As is it difficult to know whether it is the arrangement of the rooms or the culture of the care provider that influences these factors, the authors of the study have concluded that women and their partners should be informed of the benefits of furniture and equipment arrangements that support and value the physiology of birth and respect the normal functioning of the body.

Discuss with your care provider the way in which you would like to experience your pregnancy, and the various locations where you could give birth: at home, at a birthing center, or at a hospital. If you choose to give birth at a hospital, inform yourself about the non-pharmacological pain relief and comfort measures that will be available to you (continuous support, birth ball, baths, massages). Try also to learn whether the center or institution is flexible in terms of routine interventions (especially those related to movement, intermittent fetal monitoring, IV (intravenous) drip, eating and drinking, respecting your zen state, delayed cord clamping, skin to skin contact with baby, etc). Learn the rates of obstetrical interventions at the institution (e.g. inductions, cesareans, forceps, vacuum extractions, episiotomies, and epidurals).

The better you understand your needs, the better your chances are of having a satisfying birth. This is demonstrated by a study that indicates these as the four factors that impact maternal birth satisfaction: 1) attaining personal goals, 2) the quantity of support offered by care providers, 3) the quality of the relationships with the care providers, and 4) the degree of the woman's participation in decision-making[110].

COMPANIONSHIP

Attending a birth is a rich and intense experience. Because of the intensity of the sensations that the women are experiencing, companionship is necessary. The prenatal preparation that the companion has undergone influences his or her perception of the birth. For example, fathers who have prepared for their child's birth have a much more positive perception of their spouse than those who have not[111]. Women whose partners are active participants in the birth feel less pain and are more satisfied than those whose partner is not present or does not play an active role[112].

The better prepared the partner is, the more satisfying the experience will be. If, for whatever reason, the father cannot or does not wish to participate, the presence of another comforting and loving person will help you greatly. Prenatal preparation is therefore as much for the companion as it is for the mother.

In order to participate effectively, the companion should:

◆ Know how to create conditions conducive to a normal physiological birth — a birth that relies on the innate functioning of the body. He or she understands the importance of respecting a woman's zen state by creating a calm, comforting, intimate and warm atmosphere. He or she decodes the mother's stress and distress signals and supports the woman with love.
◆ Practice the techniques for modulating (or altering) pain perception: breathing (chapter 4), positions for soothing the woman during labor and birth (chapter 5), massages (chapter 6), relaxation (chapter 7) and mental imagery (chapter 8). In this way, the companion can support the mother and be a valuable resource.

Professional birth companions (doulas) provide an excellent way to support the mother and the father during all stages of labor. I recommend seeking their assistance in accompanying you throughout your birth experience.

PRACTICAL EXERCISE: GET TO KNOW THE MOTHERBABY RIGHTS
In order to guide you in your preparations for the birth, read through the Mother-Baby Rights, published by the International MotherBaby Childbirth Organization (see Appendix 3: MotherBaby Rights). In this document, you will find a description of the rights of women during pregnancy, labor and birth, and of the mother and baby after the birth. You can also consult information about birth plans, provided by the Society of Obstetricians and Gynecologists of Canada[113].

These steps will support you in making informed choices for your birth wishes; make sure you set aside time to be able to review them with your care provider.

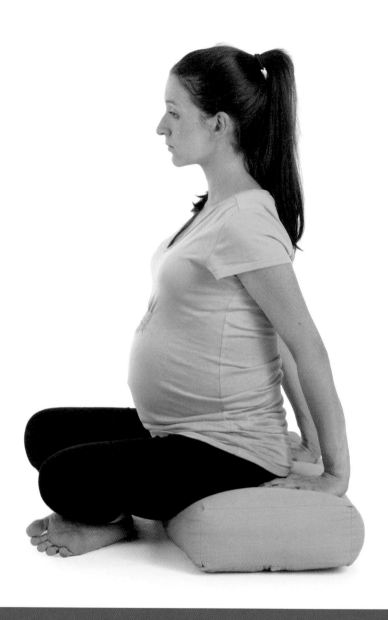

Chapter 4

BREATHING

Throughout pregnancy, conscious, slow, and deep breathing diminishes stress and anxiety, creates a calming effect and allows you to make contact with the baby growing inside you. During labor and birth, it reduces stress and strong sensations by diverting attention (third mechanism).

Breathing is a reflection of our psychological state. Short and irregular breaths indicate a state of stress and agitation, whereas slow and deep breathing translates to a state of relaxation and inner calm. Conscious breathing oxygenates the body, promotes relaxation, renews vital energy and clarifies thought.

During pregnancy, managing stress by practicing conscious, slow, and deep breathing, combined with practicing yoga poses, is beneficial for your baby. A study[114] has shown that the practice of these techniques increases the chances of bringing the pregnancy to term and reduces the risk of having a baby with a low birth weight. It is now recognized that maternal malnutrition, psychological stress or perturbed hormonal status during pregnancy can be damaging to the baby's development[115].

During rushes, paying attention to your breath will quiet the mind, calm you and help you concentrate. The repetition of key words along with your breath will help you stay in the present moment. Between rushes, your breath will help you recover and rest. During and in between rushes, observing your breath breaks the cycle of fear-tension-pain.

Summary of Chapter 4: Breathing

OBJECTIVE	METHOD
During pregnancy, recognize when you are under stress (i.e. your psychological state)	◆ Practice conscious observation of breath
During pregnancy, oxygenate the body and make contact with the baby	◆ Practice basic breathing (Ujjayi)
During labor and birth, reduce stress and strong sensations, relax and make use of periods of rest	◆ Practice basic breathing (Ujjayi) with or without chanting HU (pronounced HUE) or the sound BOA

When it comes to breathing techniques, the partner's role is essentially that of a guide. He reminds the woman to exhale deeply and to let the rush go by releasing the buttocks, the mouth and the lips.

The woman's role is to practice the breathing techniques every day, before the yoga practice session. She uses the breathing as an indicator of her state. At the birth, she exhales slowly and deeply.

BREATHING TECHNIQUES

Breathing is practiced without effort and promotes relaxation. It is an automatic function, and yet, a partial exhalation at 70% pulmonary capacity during a few respiratory cycles immediately triggers a feeling of anxiety. Slow breathing and deep exhalation create a calming effect[116].

During pregnancy and labor, slow and deep breathing will:

◆ Provide better oxygenation for mother and baby
◆ Boost the work of respiratory muscles that move the perineal diaphragm and the respiratory diaphragm
◆ Promote physical and mental relaxation
◆ Improve the mother's concentration and help her to control her mind

The Respiratory Cycle and Rhythm

Each breath is composed of a respiratory cycle which can be divided into four parts:
1. The inhalation (IN) consists of filling the lungs with air.
2. Full retention (FR) indicates the pause when the lungs are full.
3. Exhalation (EX) consists of emptying the lungs of air.
4. Empty retention (ER) indicates the pause when the lungs are empty. This is a pause that occurs naturally between the EX and the IN.

During pregnancy, I recommend that you gently inhale for a few seconds without strain and then slowly exhale. Begin each practice session with conscious and passive observation of your breathing.

Counting Breaths Using the Spiral

There is a simple method to help you concentrate on your breathing: count the breathing cycles on your fingers by drawing a spiral on the phalanges (finger bones) of your hand (*illustration 4.1*).

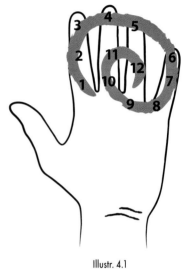

Place the thumb of your left hand on the proximal phalange (lower third) of the index finger of the same hand. Count 1 for one respiratory cycle that includes inhalation (IN) and exhalation (EX). Move the thumb onto the intermediate phalange (middle third) of the index finger to begin the next cycle. Proceed this way for a set of 12 cycles, drawing a spiral that ends on the intermediate phalange (middle third) of the ring finger.

During your labor, this spiral will help you to stay concentrated on your breathing and focus your mind. In the following paragraphs, I recommend some breathing techniques that are adapted to pregnant women.

Illustr. 4.1

Basic Breathing (Ujjayi)

Basic breathing is a simple and useful breathing technique to practice:

- During pregnancy this is used to develop your lung capacity, to relax, to recharge your energy and clear your mind
- During and between rushes this is used to stay calm, reduce stress and intense sensations by the diversion of attention (third mechanism, table 2.1)

1. Before beginning the exercise, consciously observe your breathing without changing it.
2. Exhale gently through the nose.

3. Inhale with the entire body. Imagine that the air enters through your feet. Make the air pass through your legs, your pelvis, and inflate your chest which gets bigger on the sides, in thickness, and height.
4. Observe the opening motion.
5. Observe the closing motion when exhaling through the nose.

When you inhale, the respiratory diaphragm (muscle that separates the chest cavity from the abdomen) spreads sideways, without strain, to let the lungs fill with air. When you exhale, the diaphragm relaxes, rises and empties the lungs. The perineal diaphragm (deep perineum, *illustration 1.4*) follows the movement of the respiratory diaphragm. It lowers on inhalation and rises on the exhalation. It is this movement of these diaphragms that provides relief by creating space in the abdomen for the uterus to move.

Between rushes, breathe slowly and deeply through the nose, and relax the throat. The breathing is harmonious and allows you to recover. Stay in your zen state. Listen and observe your breathing. Keep your attention on your breath. Fill up with energy. Rest.

Basic Breathing with Chanting

With this breathing technique, all the steps are the same as for basic breathing, except that the exhalation is done by the mouth rather than the nose. Chant the sound HU (pronounced HUE) or the sound BOA[117], which make the respiratory and perineal diaphragms move without effort. Thus, pressure on the uterus is lessened. Relax your buttocks, mouth and lips to keep the perineum supple.
Basic breathing with chanting is useful for long and intense rushes.

Shallow Breathing

If the urge to push arises before the cervix is fully dilated, or if you have to slow the pushing to protect your perineum, reduce pressure on the perineum by choosing buttocks-up positions (figs. 4.1 and 4.2). Do shallow exhalations and inhalations to avoid putting pressure on the uterus.

As needed, consult table 4.1, which presents a summary of breathing techniques.

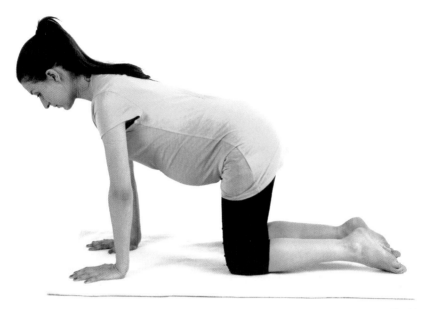

Fig. 4.1

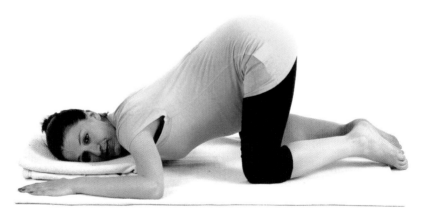

Fig. 4.2

Table 4.1 – Three Breathing Techniques

TECHNIQUE	DESCRIPTION	USAGE
Basic breathing	◆ Exhale through the nose or through the mouth during intense rushes ◆ Inhale through the nose and imagine the air entering the entire body ◆ During rushes, relax the buttocks, the mouth, and the lips	◆ To relax during daily life ◆ Between each rush ◆ Throughout labor
Basic breathing with Chanting	◆ Exhale by chanting the sound HU (pronounced HUE) or BOA during the exhalation	◆ During long and intense rushes
Shallow breathing	◆ Exhale and inhale very shallowly to avoid putting pressure on the uterus	◆ When the cervix is not fully dilated and you feel the urge to push ◆ When you want to slow the pushing to protect your perineum

Your Breathing During Pregnancy

Here are some tips to facilitate the practice of breathing techniques during pregnancy:

- Do your breathing practice at any time of day.
- Practice the breathing in supine positions: see the variations of the relaxation pose (*figure 1.31*). If you feel your back and abdominal muscles are strong enough, adopt the tall sitting pose (*figure 1.10*) or the kneeling seated pose (*figure 1.13*), both presented in chapter 1.
- Be sure to keep your back straight, to allow the respiratory diaphragm to move. Your shoulders are low and rotated back, to open the chest and unblock it. When the positioning is right, the breathing is easy.
- Never force your breath.
- If your blood pressure rises, you feel hot flashes, your face turns red, or you feel short of breath, your should reduce the duration of the inhalation and the exhalation or reduce the number of breaths. You can also stop, rest and breathe normally.

Your Breathing During the Birth

Here are some tips to facilitate the practice of breathing techniques during the birth:

- Practice the breathing techniques no matter which position you are in. If your breathing is short and irregular, make sure that your back is straight, shoulders are rotated back, and the chest is opened.

- Concentrate on your breathing to stay in touch with your sensations.
- Exhale through the nose with each rush. During intense rushes, you may feel more comfortable exhaling through the mouth.
- Make sounds, or chant the sounds HU or BOA as needed.
- Keep the mouth, tongue and buttocks soft, to relax the pelvic floor muscles.
- Adjust the breathing (length of exhalation) according to the intensity of the rush.
- Don't hold your breath, since this will only increase pressure on the uterus, and, by extension, the intensity of the sensation.
- Observe how you feel during the rushes. The breath is one of the indicators that will allow you to be aware of your sensations. If you or your partner exhibit one of the following signs of stress: pale or red face, clenched teeth and jaws, tense face, stiff hands or stretched toes, you should exhale and relax the lips, mouth and buttocks. Remember that stress hormones are contagious. The stress or relaxation levels of partners impacts the laboring woman.
- Make good use of the period in between rushes to rest. Practice slow and deep breathing.

PRACTICAL EXERCISE: OPTIMAL OXYGENATION

The following exercise is designed to help you during pregnancy and birth, as it promotes good oxygenation for you and your baby. It also develops the habit of breathing consciously in times of stress.

- Start with one set and gradually increase to two sets of 12 breaths every day, counting on your fingers (*illustration 4.1*).
- Do your breathing session before your yoga practice, or at any time during the day.
- Inhale and exhale through both nostrils, without tensing the throat. Never force your breath.
- If you feel tired, lie down and rest.

Your Breathing Session

1. Take up the relaxation pose (*figure 1.31*), the tall seated pose (*figure 1.10*) or the kneeling pose (*figure 1.13*).
2. With your eyes open, observe your breath without changing it. This is conscious breathing.

3. Close your eyes and practice the 24 basic breathing cycles. Some days, 24 breaths might make you feel agitated. Stop, rest and reduce the number of breaths.
4. After 24 breaths, observe your breathing and how you feel.
5. Write down your experience in a notebook, describing how you felt after the practice.

"At the beginning of breathing practice, I was a little agitated, with short breathing. After a few breaths, I calmed down and felt a peace spread throughout my body."

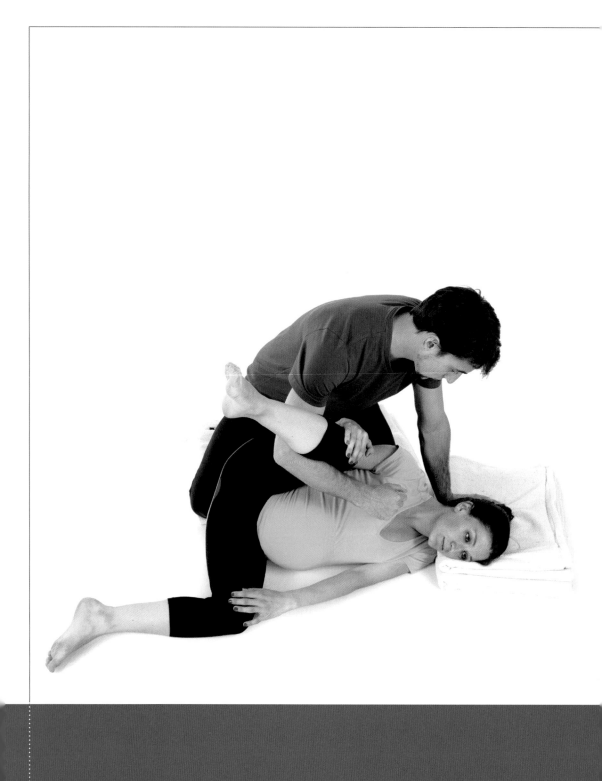

Chapter 5

MOVEMENT

The era of preventing women from moving during labor and birth is over. We now know that using different positions during labor increases the effectiveness of rushes and helps the baby's descent into the pelvis, which makes labor shorter and more pleasurable[118,119,120,121]. What is not often understood is that, in pregnancy and labor, with the release of the hormone relaxin, ligaments and pelvic joints become much more flexible. As a woman moves, this flexibility allows her to widen the diameter of her pelvis. This gives the baby more room to descend down the birth canal.

There is no universal position ideal for every woman. The positions that provide relief during labor vary from woman to woman. These relief positions also vary over the course of labor, for the same woman. The positions described in this chapter are suggestions to help you become aware of (and in tune with) your body. They are designed to relieve certain discomforts, and to encourage you to discover ways to feel good. These positions simultaneously promote your innate birth physiology – i.e. the natural functions of your body.

You can experiment with different positions throughout pregnancy and take note of the sensations and benefits that they produce. Be creative on the day of the birth and rely on your senses and your instinct. You can invent positions and movements that will provide relief and will act favorably on the progress of labor. By varying positions, you will benefit from the following:

- Better quality rushes that help the cervix to dilate;
- Facilitation of baby's positioning and descent into the pelvis;
- A reduction in your need for pain medication[122].

Summary of Chapter 5: Movement

OBJECTIVE	METHOD
Relieve the woman during all phases of labor	◆ Practice standing, seated, kneeling and supine poses that promote relaxation and the practice of massages
Optimize the physiological process of labor and birth	◆ Practice positions that promote the opening of the pelvis, the alignment and descent of the baby into the mother's pelvis
Optimize the mother's efforts during the bearing down and birthing stage	◆ Create an environment that promotes the triggering of the fetus ejection reflex ◆ Know the action to take if the fetus ejection reflex doesn't kick in
Promote the partner's active participation	◆ Partner gives continued, loving and supportive presence ◆ Partner collaborates to get mother into massage positions that promote the mother's relaxation ◆ Partner respects and protects of the woman's zen state

During labor, the companion's role is to help the woman create her zen state and stay in it. The partner can achieve this through massage and supporting her with relaxation positions. In order for the fetus ejection reflex to be activated, the companion creates a suitable environment: dimmed lights and an intimate ambience, security, and love. During the birthing of the baby, the partner has confidence in the birthing woman because they know that she has all the internal mechanisms and resources needed to bring her baby into the world safely.

The mother's role is to follow her instincts to lead her into positions that increase her comfort and promote the baby's descent. During the birth of her baby, she is vertical (squatting or kneeling). If she is exhausted, she is lying on her side, and allows the baby to descend until the fetus ejection reflex begins. Even if she is afraid, she continues to remain courageous and trust in her body and her baby.

MOVING DURING ACTIVE LABOR

Here are some tips that could help you in your search for comfort[123,124,125,126,127,128,129,131,131]. Go with what feels best:

- ◆ Follow your instinct. The intense sensations will guide you. Seek to improve your comfort, one rush at a time. Be creative, both you and your partner.
- ◆ Trust your intuition and listen for signs.
- ◆ Gaze into your partner's eyes.
- ◆ Create darkness to reduce the stimulation of your senses.
- ◆ Allow yourself some 'alone time' with your partner if that feels rights. Skin to skin contact and being intimate will increase the hormones that facilitate labor and make you feel safe.
- ◆ If you feel inclined to, kiss your partner.

- Add the poses described in chapter 1 to the poses proposed in the current chapter, since they also release tension, balance the pelvis and promote optimal descent of the baby. The objective of the positions is to make the birth more pleasurable, effective, and safe.
- Lift your arms and elongate your back to facilitate breathing.
- Alternate the angle of your feet, since opening and closing your toes increases the inner diameters of the pelvis by allowing the pelvic joints to move. This facilitates the baby's descent[132].
- Relax your abdominal muscles and legs in order to avoid tensions that increase the strong sensations of the rushes. Relax your perineum by releasing your buttocks.
- Breathe and relax your cheeks and lips.
- Let yourself go by placing all of your weight on your partner, a ball, or a prop. Imagine that you are soft inside.
- Bend forward to facilitate the optimal positioning of the baby in the uterus (the baby's back is turned toward your stomach).
- Use your yoga mat to modify your position on the floor, and use different objects to help you: cushions, balls, toilet/sink, rebozo[133] (a long and wide scarf used to carry the baby), stool, table, chairs, etc.
- Avoid positions lying on your back, as these increase back tension, restrict blood circulation due to vena cava compression (vein situated along your back that carries blood to your heart), and make the baby's descent difficult.

The Uterus Tilts Forward During Rushes

If, after a few minutes, you notice that your position is not providing relief or that the baby is not descending, experiment with other positions, knowing that none of them will reduce the sensations you feel completely. If you have an electronic fetal heart monitor, keep moving while making sure to stabilize the sensor. As needed, your companion can reposition it, maintaining it in the same place on your stomach, so that the device can record the data.

Moving during labor has numerous benefits. The first is that it helps the cervix dilate. Under the effect of the rush, the uterus tilts forward. When you

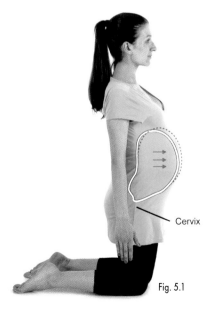

Cervix

Fig. 5.1

are in a standing position, back straight, the uterus does not have to fight against gravity (*figure 5.1*).

When you are lying on your back (*figure 5.2*) or semi-reclined, the uterus has to work against gravity to tilt forward[134].

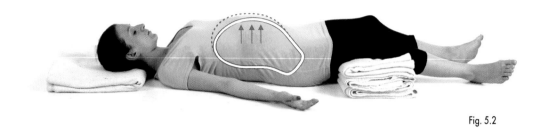

Fig. 5.2

THE UTERUS WORKS AGAINST GRAVITY TO TILT FORWARD

When your back is leaning forward, the uterus benefits from gravity, which helps it tilt forward (*figure 5.3*).

GRAVITY HELPS THE UTERUS TO TILT FORWARD

Using a Ball

Balls started to be used in maternity wards at the beginning of the 1990s. Simple and inexpensive, they offer many advantages that women appreciate during labor. To make full use of the ball, be sure to take the following precautions:

- Make sure that your ball is clean.
- Place a blanket, mat or towel under the ball to keep it clean.

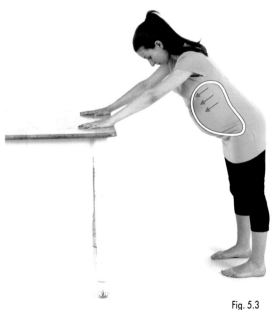

Fig. 5.3

- Before sitting on the ball, make sure to cover it with a towel that you can change as needed.
- Stabilize the ball so that you feel secure, by supporting yourself with your partner, a wall, or a chair, for example.
- Ask your partner for help getting on and off of the ball.
- Choose the right size ball. Generally speaking, when you are sitting on the ball, your calf and thigh should form a 90 degree angle.

Give your imagination full freedom and use the ball in different ways, for example:

- To massage your back, by placing it between yourself and a wall;
- To support your upper body, by placing it in front of you;
- To stretch your side, by placing it next to you;
- To arch your back, by resting your back on it.

Different Positions to Facilitate Active Labor

All the positions described in the following paragraphs aim to provide you with relief during active labor. Trust this process, it may take courage, but your efforts will be rewarded.

STANDING POSITION, SUPPORTED BY A WALL, YOUR PARTNER, OR A BALL

Four standing positions are proposed here.

STEPS

1. Standing, with your forehead against the wall, fold your arms over your head (*figure 5.4*). Alternate the angle of your feet. Gently rock your pelvis to the right and then to the left.
2. A variation is to use your partner for support (*figure 5.5*). When you release your legs, your back lengthens, which provides additional relief (*figure 5.6*).
3. Standing, with your upper body supported by a ball that is placed on a table, a bed, or against a wall, extend your arms (*figure 5.7*). Alternate the angle of your feet to increase the inner diameters of the pelvis by allowing the pelvic joints to move. Rock your pelvis gently to the right and then to the left. This position helps your baby descend.

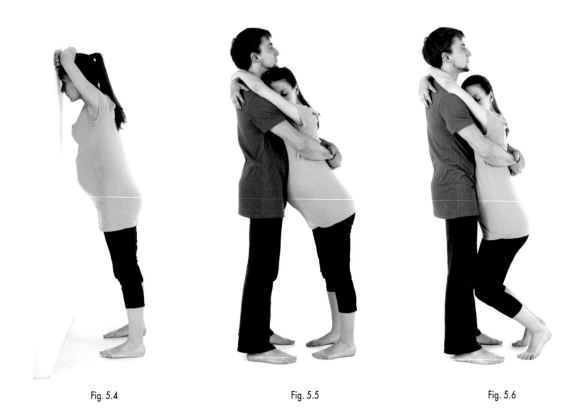

Fig. 5.4   Fig. 5.5   Fig. 5.6

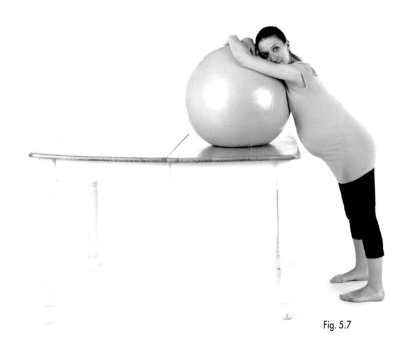

Fig. 5.7

TRUSTING BIRTH WITH THE BONAPACE METHOD

HALF-STANDING, HALF-SEATED POSITION, SUPPORTED BY A WALL

The following position allows your perineum to relax.

Sit on your partner's thigh, with your partner standing behind you (*figure 5.8*).

STEPS

1. Rest your upper body against the wall in front of you and lift your arms above your head.
2. Relax your abdominal muscles, your legs, buttocks and deep perineum. Imagine that you are soft inside.
3. Move the pelvis by following the light movements of your partner's thigh.

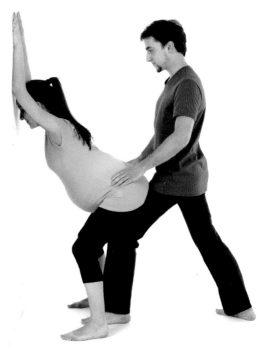

Fig. 5.8

KNEELING, FORWARD-LEANING POSITION

The following five positions are effective for back relief and massage. Find comfort by adjusting the height of the support under your arms, by placing your perineum on your partner or on a semi-rigid cushion, by placing a blanket between your heels and buttocks, or by placing one foot on the floor, to create a semi-sitting, semi-squatting position. Your partner uses a rebozo to support and cradle your belly.

STEPS

1. By placing a blanket over your heels and underneath your buttocks, you reduce the pressure on the ankles (*figure 5.9*). Applying pressure on the lower back lengthens it and relieves tensions.
2. Rest the upper body on a chair for more height (*figure 5.10*). By placing one foot on the floor, so that you are half kneeling and half squatting, you create an asymmetry that opens the pelvis.

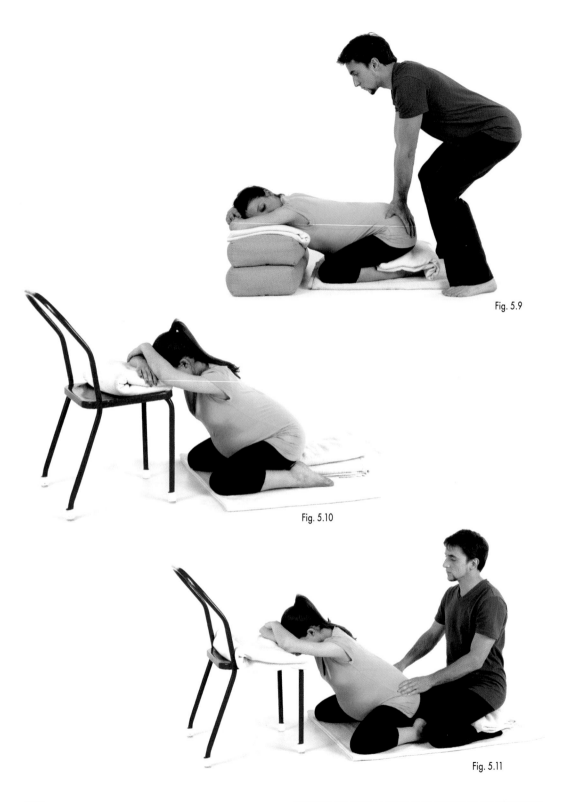

Fig. 5.9

Fig. 5.10

Fig. 5.11

TRUSTING BIRTH WITH THE BONAPACE METHOD

3. Another way to reduce pressure on the ankles and legs is to rest the perineum on a support or on your partner's knee (*figure 5.11*).
4. A rebozo is an excellent tool to relieve back tension (*figure 5.12*). After the birth, it can also be used to carry your baby.
5. During intense rushes, rest the forearms on the floor and relax the head and buttocks. The rebozo helps create a soothing traction in the pelvis (*figure 5.13*).

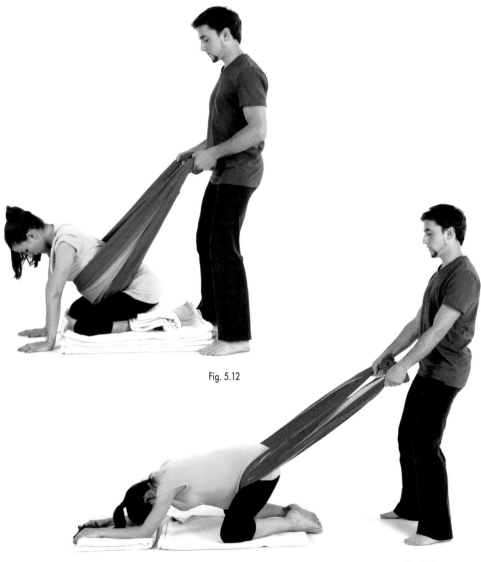

Fig. 5.12

Fig. 5.13

I recommend the following three positions seated on a ball.

STEPS

1. Sitting on a ball with your toes close to the wall, lengthen your back and open the chest by pressing the elbows against the wall (*figure 5.14*).

2. Support the upper body on a table (*figure 5.15*). Relax the buttocks by balancing on the ball and have someone massage your lower back.

3. Between rushes, rest by leaning on your partner (*figure 5.16*).

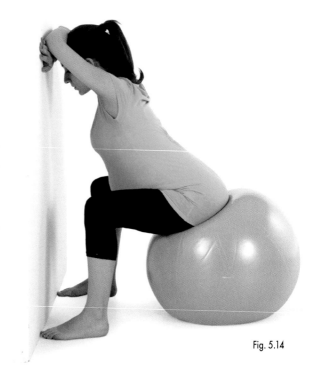

Fig. 5.14

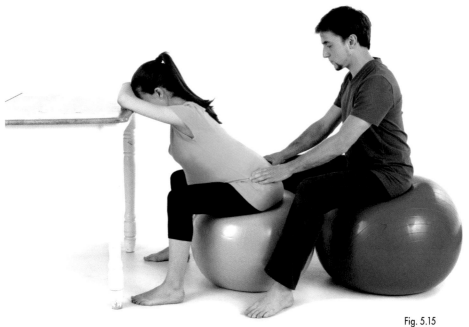

Fig. 5.15

Beneficial Effects:

- Your back is tilted forward. Thus, your uterus benefits from gravity, which helps it to move and dilate.
- Your arms are elevated and your back is lengthened, which facilitates breathing.
- Your baby moves in the pelvis thanks to small hip movements.

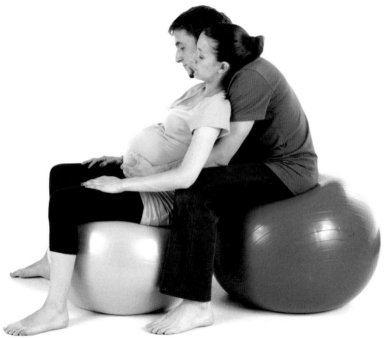

Fig. 5.16

SQUATTING POSITION WITH ARMS SUSPENDED

The squatting position with your arms suspended can promote your baby's descent. This position is made easier using the rebozo, which helps lengthen your back. Changing the angle of your feet increases the inner diameters of the pelvis. When your baby is high, turning your toes outwards will increase the diameter of the pelvic inlet (upper part of your pelvis) to facilitate the baby's entry into the pelvis. Your sit bones will come closer. When the baby is low and descending (bearing down and birthing stage), place your feet parallel to open the pelvic outlet (lower part of your pelvis). Your sit bones will spread apart. Three options are presented.

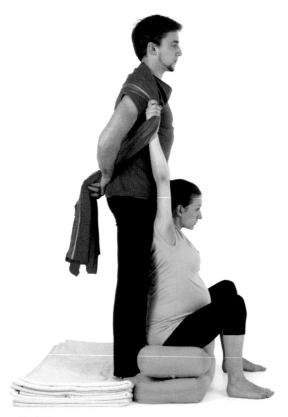

Fig. 5.17

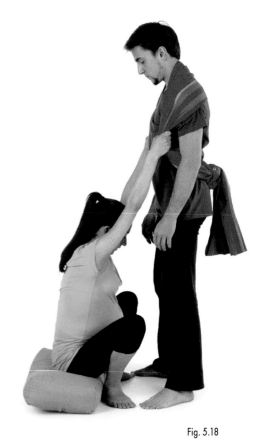

Fig. 5.18

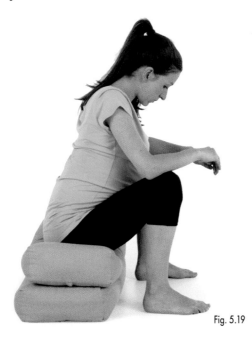

Fig. 5.19

STEPS

1. Lengthen your back with the help of your partner, who is behind you (*figure 5.17*). To protect your partner's neck, make sure that the rebozo is behind their shoulders.
2. Position yourself facing your partner (*figure 5.18*).
3. Take the squatting position, sitting on semi-rigid supports, arms pressed against the knees (*figure 5.19*).

TRUSTING BIRTH WITH THE BONAPACE METHOD

Another way to reap the benefits of the squatting position is to suspend yourself between the legs of your partner who is sitting on a high stool, a table, or a bed. His feet rest on lower chairs, positioned at your sitting level[135] (*figure 5.20*).

Beneficial Effects:
- Rushes are stronger and more frequent[136,137].
- The diameter of the pelvis increases.
- Gravity promotes the baby's descent.

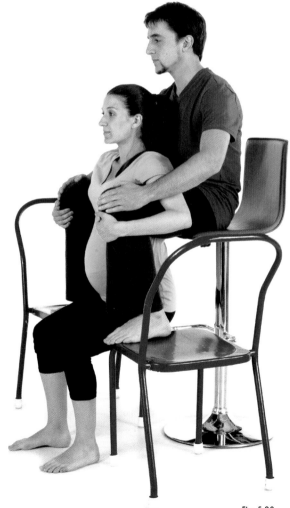

Fig. 5.20

During the examination in which labor's progress is measured (e.g. vaginal examinations), your partner supports the weight of your legs so that you can relax your abdominal muscles, legs and buttocks (*figure 5.21*). When your knees are supported in this way, the adductors (inner thigh muscles) and perineum relax, which decreases the discomfort of rushes.

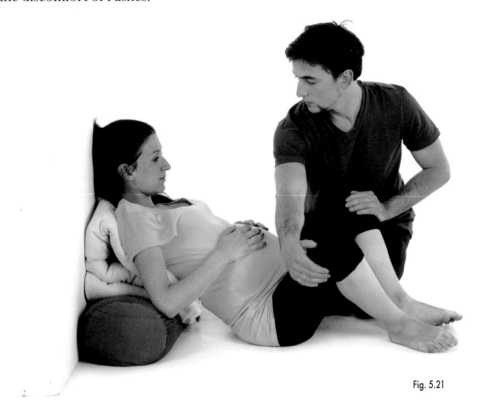

Fig. 5.21

SIDE-LYING POSITION

Lying down, preferably on your left side, head supported by a pillow, bend your right knee and put it on another pillow. Your left arm is in front of you. When the bent leg approaches your chest (*figure 5.22*), your body is in an asymmetric position, which helps the baby engage and descend into your pelvis. Make use of this position by having your lower back massaged, and by resting. Every once in a while, switch to your right side.

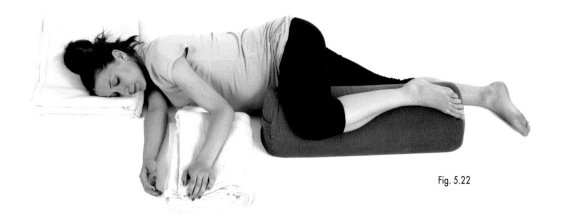

Fig. 5.22

Two Positions to Prevent Pushing

It sometimes happens that a woman feels the urge to push[138] before the cervix has completely dilated. To counter this urge, practice shallow breathing and take up one of the two following positions:

CLOSED POSITION, LYING ON THE STOMACH

The closed position, lying on the stomach (*figure 5.23*) decreases pressure on the perineum, which helps you to not push prematurely. Relax the buttocks completely.

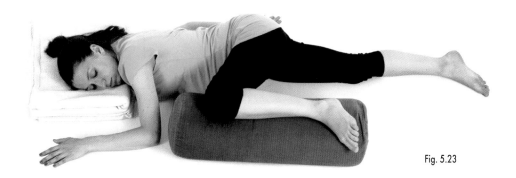

Fig. 5.23

The kneeling position, supported on lower arms, can be used when the urge to push is felt before complete dilation, or when the baby's descent does not seem to be progressing. This sometimes occurs when the baby is in the occiput posterior position (*illustration 1.11*), with his back toward yours. In this position, the mother can bend forward and position her shoulders close to the floor, below her pelvis. Gravity disengages the baby's head from the pelvis and allows the baby to adjust to a better position to enter the pelvis (*figure 5.24*). However, this position should not be used if your baby is not yet engaged in the pelvis.

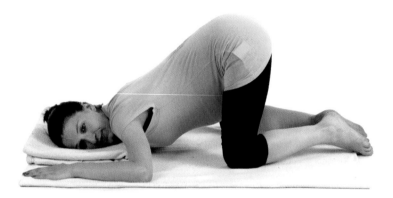

Fig. 5.24

Beneficial Effects:
- The pressure of your baby on the cervix is lessened, which can help you hold back when the urge to push is strong.
- Pressure on hemorrhoids is reduced.

Three Positions for Turning an Occiput Posterior Baby

When your baby is in the occiput posterior position (*illustration 1.11*), with baby's back towards your back, and its face towards your belly, labor complications may be increased. To help turn the baby's back to the front of your belly, do not stay on your back. The uterus has to work very hard to rotate the baby and the baby's oxygenation is not very good due to compression of the vena cava (vein situated along your back that carries blood to your heart). It is best to practice the following three positions.

KNEELING POSITION WITH PELVIC TRACTION

A variation on the preceding position involves applying traction on the pelvis with a rebozo, to lengthen and soothe the back (*figure 5.25*).

SEMI-LYING POSITION WITH BENT LEG

Semi-lying on your left side to promote blood circulation, bend and lift your upper leg (*figure 5.26*). Direct your partner to support your lifted right leg. Switch sides and extend the lower leg to adjust the angles of your pelvis opening.

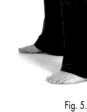

Fig. 5.25

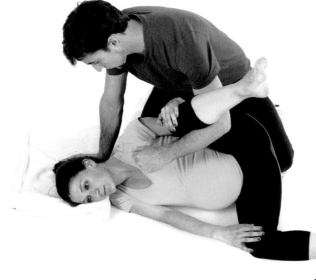

Fig. 5.26

When practiced in alternation with the closed position, lying facing down with supports (*figure 5.23*), this position helps to modify the baby's positioning.

POSITION ON ALL FOURS WITH TWO BALLS

If the baby is in the occiput posterior position, you can take up a position on all fours or leaning forward, with the stomach relaxed. Use two balls to help you keep the position (*figure 5.27*). The gravity will help to turn the baby's back, which is heavy, toward the front of your belly. The people who are accompanying you must ensure your safety and stability in this position. Cushions can be positioned to support the weight of your lower legs.

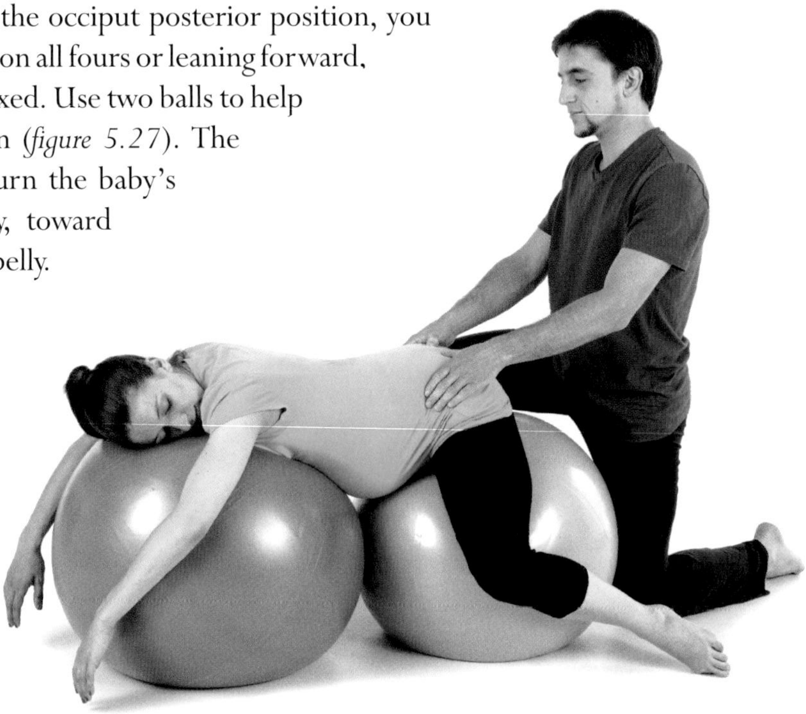

Fig. 5.27

Beneficial Effects:
- ◆ Allows the mother to rest between rushes.
- ◆ Relieves hemorrhoids.
- ◆ Is adapted for women with an epidural.
- ◆ Can slow down a second (pushing) stage that progresses very quickly.

POSITIONS FOR BIRTHING THE BABY

The way in which babies have been born has varied from one civilization to the next. For a few centuries now, in the West, women have been made to give birth lying on their backs, or semi-reclining. They have been encouraged to block their breaths and push with the abdominal muscles, as they are instructed. This reclining position is usually accompanied by the "block-push" breathing, often practiced as soon as the cervix is completely dilated, whether or not the mother feels the urge to push. The diaphragm is lowered, because of the air filling the lungs, and the rectus abdominis (abdominals) are contracted because the mother's head is lifted. This downward pressure is exerted not only on the baby, but on the uterus and bladder as well.

If it is prolonged, this pushing can cause injury to the perineal muscles and pull the ligaments that hold the organs. Urinary incontinence can result, as well as a weakening of the anal sphincter, and a slipping down of the uterus or the bladder[139].

This method of pushing provokes other negative effects, notably a drop in the mother's blood pressure, and a lack of oxygen in the baby, which can lead to deceleration of baby's heart[140]. A meta-analysis of positions during the second stage of labor, published in 2012, reveals that the use of instruments (forceps and vacuum extraction) and the frequency of episiotomy are reduced[141] for women without epidural who give birth in a vertical position, when compared with those who give birth lying on their backs.

Practices supporting the ejection of the baby are being adapted at a snail's pace worldwide, despite growing scientific evidence that confirms the negative effects of the traditional reclining position and directed pushing (Valsalva maneuver)[142,143,144,145,146].

In 1884, the American professor of obstetrics, Dr. George Engelmann (1843-1903), published an ethnographic work[147] comparing childbirth labor practices of "civilized peoples" with those of people who "let themselves be governed by their instincts". What follows is the outcome of his study.

In those who are governed by their instincts:

- The woman's culture, tradition and the shape of her pelvis determine whether she gives birth standing, kneeling, or lying facing downward;
- The positions she adopts differ according to the stage of labor;
- The woman avoids the position of lying on her back, especially at the end of labor.

In "civilized" people:

- The lying-on-the-back position that is taught in obstetrics is one of the "fashions" that do not seem to respect the laboring woman's nature;
- In this position, the woman has to make great efforts to push her baby out, since the baby has to forge a path while fighting against gravity;
- The process of labor is prolonged, and is less safe, efficient, and pleasant.

Like many researchers[148], Dr. Engelmann concluded that there is no reason to restrict women to giving birth lying on their backs. Following one's instinct is demonstrably a more effective way to give birth.

Reference the illustrations 5.1 to 5.6: published in Professor Engelmann's work. They represent 19th Century childbirth scenes from people governed by their instincts. None of the women are on their backs and, even then, men were supporting the women in birth. These images will inspire your imagination for the bearing down and birthing stage.

The Fetus Ejection Reflex

In 1957, Dr. Constance Beynon[149], a British obstetrician, published the results of observations she collected in a context where the birthing woman is allowed to freely follow her instinct:

- The strong, involuntary and irresistible pushing happens when the baby presses on the pelvic floor. This mechanism is similar to that of defecation.
- There is a brief interval between the beginning of a rush and the involuntary push.
- The irresistible urge to push varies from one rush to another.

Dr. Beynon proposes that, rather than hurrying the woman to birth the baby by telling her to push, it would be preferable to encourage her to take her time and push gently, when the urge to push is irresistible. In chapter 3, we saw that the Ferguson reflex and the fetus ejection reflex are activated when the conditions are favorable. Such optimal conditions include:

- Creating an environment (tranquil, dimmed lighting, warm, intimate) where the birthing woman feels secure and protected.
- Avoiding stimulation of the woman's cortex or the thinking brain (by disturbing and overstimulating the woman by talking or asking her questions that require her to think).
- Allowing the baby to activate the pelvic floor receptors, which will give the signal to the brain to send out more oxytocin, which will provoke powerful rushes that will aid the baby in descending further. Pushing too early is detrimental to the activation of the fetus ejection reflex[150,151].

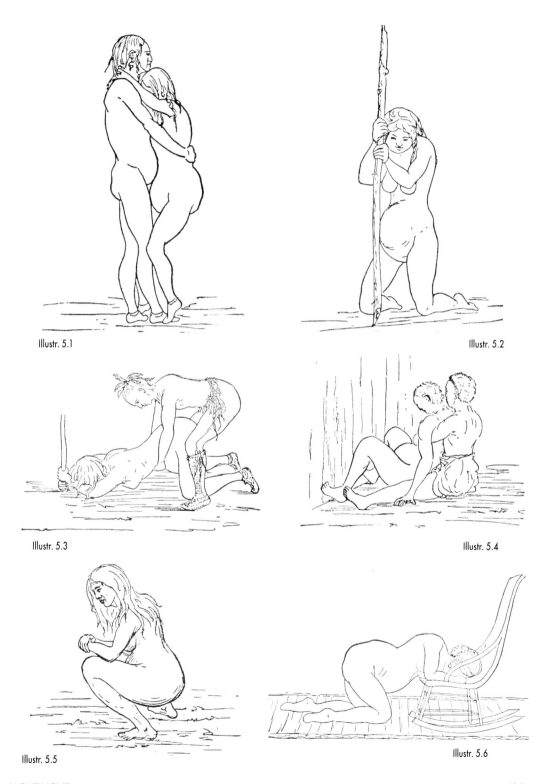

Illustr. 5.1

Illustr. 5.2

Illustr. 5.3

Illustr. 5.4

Illustr. 5.5

Illustr. 5.6

In order to prepare for establishing the conditions that encourage the activation of the fetus ejection reflex:

- Speak with the care provider that you've chosen to accompany you during your pregnancy about the ways you wish to birth your baby.
- Write down your birth wishes in a document that you will give to those who will be present at your birth.
- Protect your zen zone – an atmosphere that allows you to access your instincts.

When the reflex has been activated, all you need to do is allow yourself to be guided by the pushing. During each push, imagine the vagina opening. Imagine opening the passage for the baby. Concentrate your energy on the baby's descent.

The sequence[152] described in the next section can be used if the fetus ejection reflex does not occur, or if you have to push voluntarily to birth your baby.

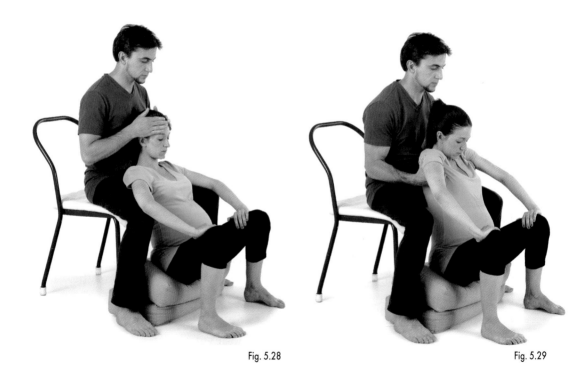

Fig. 5.28   Fig. 5.29

STEPS

1. Take up a squatting position on semi-rigid supports (*figure 5.28*). You are leaning on your partner who is sitting on a chair behind you.

2. When the rush starts, close your eyes, tuck in your chin and press your hands against your knees (*figure 5.29*). Push gently. You never want to hold your breath any longer than 5 seconds[153].

3. Between rushes, lean on your partner and rest (*figure 5.28*).

4. Follow your baby's progress by touching his head when it presents itself at the vulva (*figure 5.30*). Know that you can be the one who catches your baby at the moment of birth, and one day be able to share such a profound story with your child.

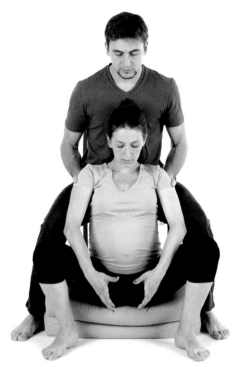

Fig. 5.30

Protecting the Perineum

Positioning and breathing during childbirth will have an impact on your perineum. A short, spontaneous push is less damaging than a long, blocked push[154,155].

Here are some practical tips for protecting your perineum.

- Practice daily yoga sessions to make your pelvic floor muscles supple and strong.
- Practice perineal massage during pregnancy[156].
- Do your best to help turn a posterior baby (*figures 5.25, 5.26 and 5.27*).
- Create an environment that is optimal for activating the ejection reflex[157,158] (dimmed lights, feeling of security, respect for your intimacy).
- Practice vertical positions (kneeling or squatting) or lying on your side[159].
- Take your time and practice patience throughout your labor[160].
- Do not hold your breath for long periods[161].
- Visualize your vagina and perineum opening to let your baby through, and relax your buttocks and your mouth.
- Use your hands to feel when the baby's head is about to come through.

- Allow yourself to make sounds[162] that encourage the respiratory and perineal diaphragm muscles to rise.

PRACTICAL EXERCISE: FILMS TO WATCH OR RE-WATCH

Our perception of birth is influenced by Hollywood movies: medicalized births, women lying on their backs, screaming, out of control, no pleasure, no power. You may notice that women around you often give birth with an epidural and find it difficult to understand why you would do differently.

In order to inform yourself about the effectiveness of alternatives and feed your imagination with positive images related to birth, watch films in which women experience their births fully, using their own internal mechanisms and resources. Here are some suggestions for films you could watch:

- Birth Day[163]
- Orgasmic Birth[164]
- Birth As We Know It[165]

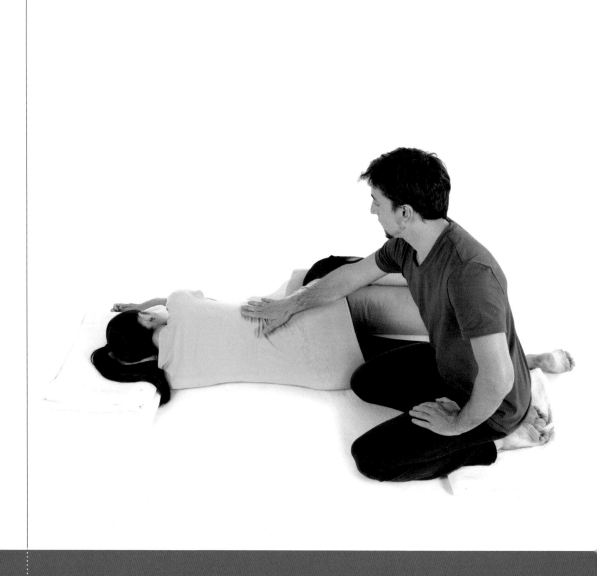

Chapter 6

MASSAGE

The benefits of massage are well-known. Practiced during labor, they give the woman relief and help to prevent difficult births.

This chapter is about two mechanisms that aim to reduce intense sensations: the first is applying a non-painful stimulation on the painful site (e.g. stroking the abdomen, or giving a light massage to relieve back pain); the second is applying a painful stimulation to a zone sometimes far away from the painful zone (e.g. massaging different acupuncture reflex zones).

The basic principles for giving a massage are always the same:

- **During pregnancy and between rushes**, in a gentle or non-painful manner, the person giving the massage strokes the painful areas to relieve or relax the pregnant woman.
- **During rushes**, the person giving the massage creates a firm and painful pressure on the acupuncture reflex zones of the woman in labor.

Besides modifying the perception of sensations, massaging acupressure zones allows for therapeutic results specific to each reflex zone. These results notably include:

- A stimulation of labor, due to efficient and quality rushes that assist your baby in descending through the birth canal;
- A reduction in the duration of labor, due to the acceleration of cervical dilation;
- Relief of lumbar pain[166, 167, 168, 169, 170].

Painful massage works on the modulation of strong sensations (e.g. rushes as well as on the progression of labor and birth).

Summary of Chapter 6: Massage

OBJECTIVE	METHOD
Modulate pain in order to provide the woman with relief	• Practice non-painful massages during pregnancy and between rushes • Practice painful massages of a reflex zone during rushes
Facilitate physiological birth (one that respects and relies on the innate functioning of the body)	• Practice painful massages on acupuncture reflex zones
Promote the participation of the partner in his role supporting the mother	• Know massages that modulate pain and prevent complicated births

The role of the companion is to apply the pain modulation techniques as well as practice painful and non-painful massages on the acupuncture reflex zones.

The role of the woman is to have confidence in the process of birth and in the effectiveness of massages in reducing her perception of strong sensations.

NON-PAINFUL MASSAGE

The virtues of relaxing massage are well-known: it reduces stress, releases muscle and nerve tensions, and irrigates the tissues. During pregnancy and between rushes, facial massage helps you to create and stay in your zen state.

Facial Massage

The face has more than 80 muscles, which are responsible for expressing emotions. Tensions appear particularly on the forehead, temples, and jaw. Light stimulation is enough to relieve tension.

Practice this massage during pregnancy and between rushes. At the beginning of the massage, brush lightly with your fingers, and then go more deeply. Moisturizing cream is preferable than oil for most people. Follow your instinct, and the tension will disappear.

1. While the woman is lying down on her back, place both of your hands under her head and find support under the bone at the base of her skull. Apply a firm and pulsating pressure for 10 seconds. Release for a few seconds and then repeat. Use this pause to gently stroke back her hair and head (*figure 6.1*).

2. Place your thumbs on her forehead and trace lines by sliding your thumbs to her temples. Make three lines at different heights. Maintain firm pressure (*figure 6.2*).
3. Pinch her eyebrows between your thumbs and index fingers. Start at the bridge of the nose, sliding along until you finish at the outer corner of her eyes. Apply light pressure and pay attention to the upper edge of the orbital bone (the bone around the eye socket). Applying firm pressure, you will feel three cavities (*figure 6.3*).
4. With the pads of your index and middle fingers, make small circles all around her temples. Alternate the direction of rotation. Apply light pressure (*figure 6.4*).
5. Lower your fingertips to follow her cheekbone, applying firm pressure, without pressing on the nostrils. Do both sides at the same time (*figure 6.5*).

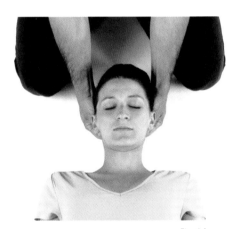

Fig. 6.1

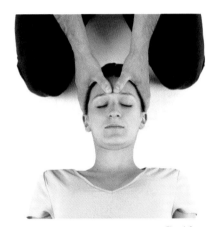

Fig. 6.2

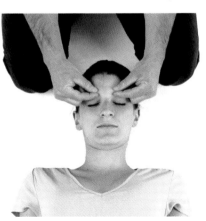

Fig. 6.3

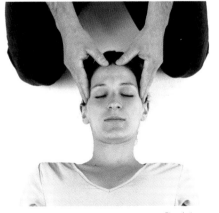

Fig. 6.4

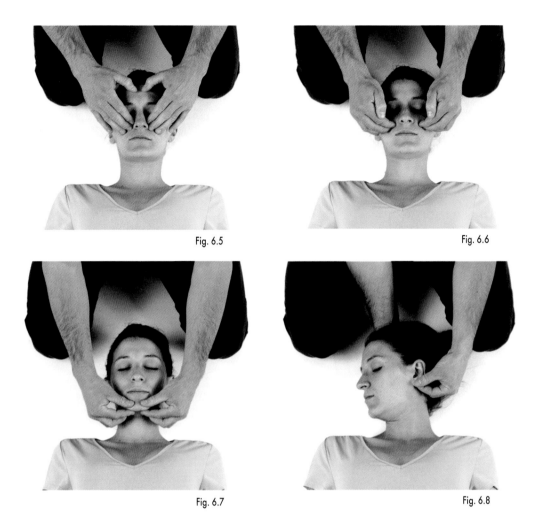

Fig. 6.5

Fig. 6.6

Fig. 6.7

Fig. 6.8

6. Gently lift her cheekbones by placing your index and middle fingers under it. Start at the bridge of the nose and move outwards until you finish on the side of her face, at the jaw joint (*figure 6.6*).

7. Join both your hands at the center of her chin and gently pinch the jawbone between your thumb and all the other fingers together. Let the hands slide all the way toward her jaw joints (*figure 6.7*).

8. Turn her head to the side. Massage her ear by pinching the lobe between your index finger and thumb. Start at the base of the ear and continue to the top. Repeat on both sides. Using your index finger and thumb, follow the edge of the ear by applying a firm pressure on the bone behind it (*figure 6.8*).

9. With the fingers, make circles all along the nape of the neck. Start at the shoulders, continuing all the way to the bone behind the ear (*figure 6.9*).

Beneficial Effects:
- ◆ Eliminates tension.
- ◆ Secures and calms the person being massaged.

Massage of the Sacrum

The sacrum (the bone at the base of your spine) harbors a large portion of lower back tension. During the birth, it must move to let the baby pass.
A simple, non-painful pressure on this zone helps to reduce discomfort.

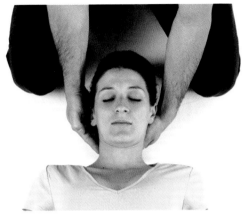

Fig. 6.9

1. Move your hands down the length of the spine, up to the separation of her buttocks.
2. Place your hands one on top of the other, fingers pointing toward the head (*figure 6.10*).

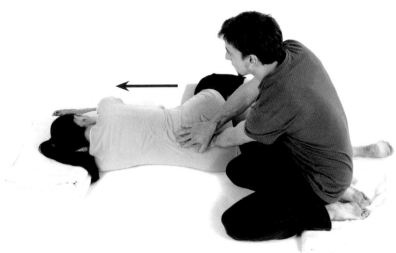

Fig. 6.10

3. **During rushes**, apply non-painful pressure to the sacrum, without moving. If you pay attention, you can feel the sacrum vibrating.
4. **Between rushes**, rub the sacrum with the palm of your hand, in an upward movement only. This helps disperse the tension in the sacrum.

Beneficial Effects:
Soothes the lower back by stabilizing the sacrum, which vibrates due to the rushes.

Massaging the Hips
Massaging the hips serves to relax tension accumulated in the psoas, a muscle that starts in the hip and attaches to the lumbar vertebrae (the spinal discs in your lower back). Since this muscle is in contact with the respiratory diaphragm, it reacts to emotional stress, particularly stress related to fear.

During pregnancy and between rushes, oil the hips. Use oils that are pleasant to the woman, including non-scented carrier oils.

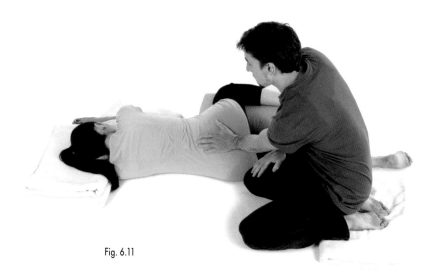

Fig. 6.11

1. Starting at the sacrum, apply pressure as you go around the hip with your hand and release the pressure once your hand has arrived at the sides and belly (*figures 6.11, 6.12 and 6.13*).
2. Reverse the direction of your stroke, putting light pressure on the sacrum as you return.

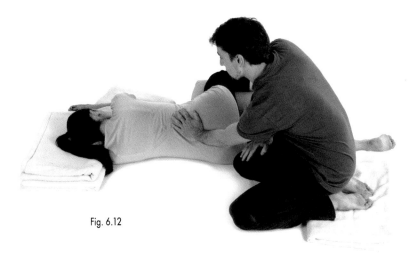

Fig. 6.12

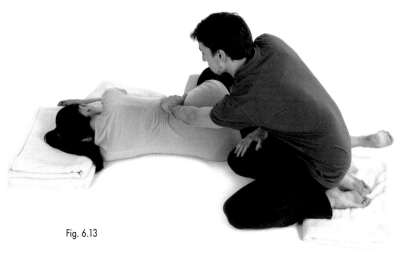

Fig. 6.13

Beneficial Effects:

Provides relief and relaxes the psoas muscles, as well as back
muscles frequently made taut during pregnancy.

Buttock Muscle Massage (G.B.-30 - Huantiao)

Acupuncture point G.B.-30 is situated in the buttock. It is at the intersection of two muscles in your buttocks: the obturator internus and the inferior gemellis. These muscles connect the pelvis at the upper edge of the greater trochanter (highest part of the femur bone in your thigh) (*illustration 6.1*).

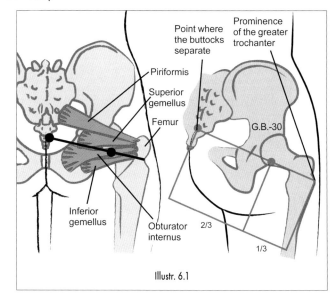

Illustr. 6.1

1. Move your hand, flattened, upward along the side of her upper leg, until you feel something protruding at the highest point of the femur bone (the greater trochanter). Place a finger just above this bump.

2. Imagine the place where the buttocks separate, and, at that point, place one finger of your opposite hand.

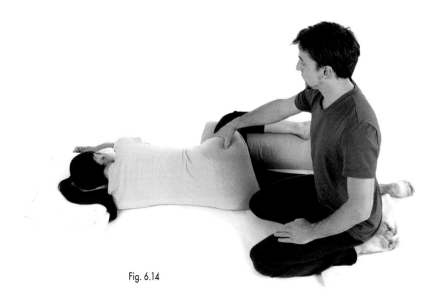

Fig. 6.14

3. Trace a line between these two points and separate it into three equal parts.
4. The point that corresponds to the first third near the protruding greater trochanter is the piriformis muscle. You will feel a numbness or an electrical charge when you apply pressure here.
5. **During pregnancy and between rushes**, apply continuous pressure to point G.B.-30 for 7 or 8 seconds, then let go (*figure 6.14*).

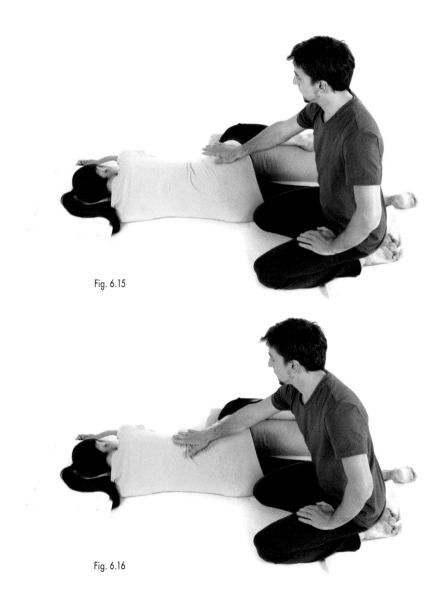

Fig. 6.15

Fig. 6.16

6. **During labor, particularly between rushes**, sweep with the palm of your hand, from the buttock muscle (*figure 6.15*) upward toward the ribs (*figure 6.16*), and from the buttock muscle (*figure 6.17*) along the leg (*figure 6.18*).

Beneficial Effects:

Relieves tension of the lower back and of the legs.

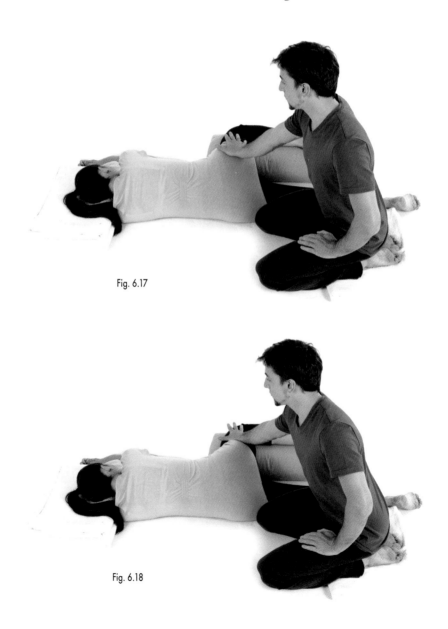

Fig. 6.17

Fig. 6.18

         TRUSTING BIRTH WITH THE BONAPACE METHOD

PAINFUL MASSAGE

The second pain modulation mechanism requires that you produce a second pain, anywhere on the body. This stimulates the release of natural morphine (endorphins), which will lessen the sensation of pain everywhere in the body, except in the zone where this second pain is being produced.

Rather than apply the secondary painful stimulation randomly, I recommend that you target acupuncture reflex zones that are recognized for their benefits during birth[171, 172, 173]. In this way, not only will you reap the benefits of the second pain, namely the release of endorphins, but also the therapeutic effects associated with acupressure.

According to the ancient science of acupuncture, the body contains a network of energy circuits called "meridians". There are also points called 'acupuncture reflex zones' where energy can be mobilized to correct health issues (*illustration 6.2*). Each meridian is associated with an organ, and bears its name: bladder (BL), large intestine (L.I.), liver (LIV), gall bladder (G.B.), etc. There are 14 principal meridians in acupuncture.

ACUPUNCTURE REFLEX ZONES

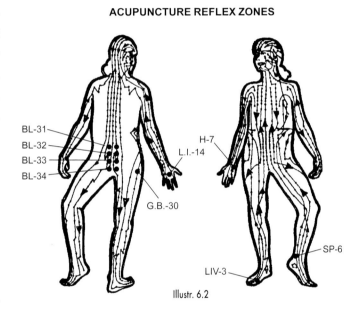

Illustr. 6.2

Some care providers use acupuncture during birth to reduce complications that are sometimes associated with birth. They facilitate the process of birth, and prevent difficulties such as the decrease in frequency and intensity of rushes, descent, and inefficient positioning of the baby, etc. It is likely that the medical professional (i.e. the person trained in acupuncture) will insert the needles in the same points that are presented below. In that case, create a second pain anywhere else on the body.

Here are some tips to help you find and use these points.

◆ They are all situated in a hollow, frequently next to a bone.

- When they are stimulated via acupressure, the subject feels a numbness or a feeling of electric shock.
- They work together to create efficient rushes, and to facilitate cervical dilation.
- The points must be stimulated in alternation, one side of the body and then the other.
- The stimulation must be painful and last the entirety of a rush.

Caution: With the exception of point G.B.-30 in the buttock, the practice of deep massage is inadvisable during pregnancy, because these points can provoke rushes.

Stimulation of the Gall Bladder, or Point G.B.-30-Huantiao

Painful stimulation of G.B.-30 during a rush modulates (or alters) all the pain in the body except for the point G.B.-30 itself.

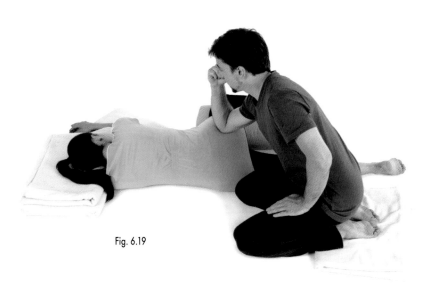

Fig. 6.19

Painful pressure can be created on this point by using a finger or an elbow. During rushes, apply strong, painful pressure that lasts for the entire rush.

Beneficial Effects:

Relieves tension in the lower back and legs.

Stimulation of the Bladder, or Points BL-31 to BL-34

Points BL-31 to BL-34 are situated in the sacrum, and correspond to the eight (i.e. two sets of four) holes of this bone. These points are the basis of multiple birth-related acupuncture treatments, as they have an effect on rushes. However, they can sometimes be difficult to locate.

Before starting the painful massage, you need to find points BL-31 to BL-34. To do this, draw an imaginary triangle on the sacrum to visualize the zone that contains these four points. Here is how to find them:

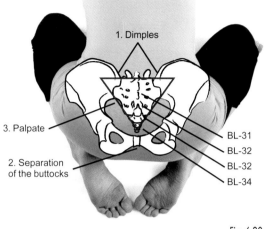

Fig. 6.20

1. Draw the line at the top of the triangle. It is at the same height as the two dimples, which are situated below and to either side of the spine (*figure 6.20*).
2. Place a point where the buttocks separate. This is the tip of the triangle.

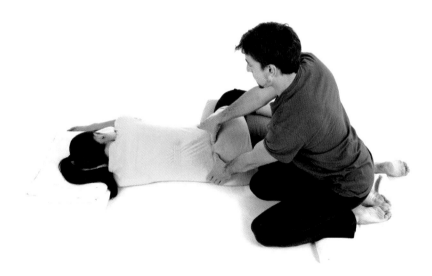

Fig. 6.21

3. Define the size of the triangle by feeling for the sides of the sacrum (the bone at the base of the spine). Draw two lines that complete the triangle.
4. Inside the triangle are the points BL-31 to BL-34. They are in a row of four, one below the other, and at the same height on both sides of the spine. The distance between the two rows is the same as the width of the spine.

During pregnancy, massage these points with the palm of the hand only, non-painfully, since these points can stimulate rushes (*figure 6.21*).

During rushes, apply strong, painful pressure for the entire rush.

Start with BL-31 (the uppermost points) by massaging both sides at once, and continue with points BL-32, BL-33, and BL-34.

Beneficial Effects:
- Works with the other acupuncture reflex zones to help induce and stimulate labor.
- Relieves back pain during rushes.

Stimulating the large intestine, or point L.I.-4-Hegu

Point L.I.-4 is frequently used in self-defense classes. It is very effective, due to its easy access and the pain it provokes.

1. Before starting the painful massage, you have to find point L.I.-4.
2. To do so, follow the index finger downward, starting from its tip. You will find a small cavity near the meeting-point of the metacarpals (the bones beneath the back of the hand) of the index finger and thumb (*illustration 6.3*). Use your

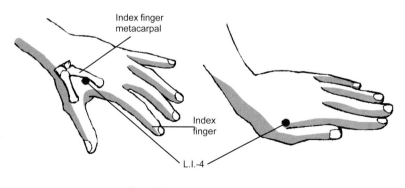

Index finger metacarpal

Index finger

L.I.-4

Illustr. 6.3

index finger and thumb to pinch the spot halfway between the index finger knuckle and the wrist joint, alongside the index finger's metacarpal.

3. **During rushes**, apply firm and painful pressure to this point.

Beneficial Effects:

- Works with the other acupuncture reflex zones to help induce and stimulate labor.
- Facilitates the descent of the baby in the birth canal during the second stage of labor.

Stimulating the liver, or point LIV-3-Taichong

Point LIV-3 is easily accessible during rushes. However, some women do not feel strong sensations from the stimulation of this point. In this case, opt for other points.

1. Before applying painful pressure, you have to find point LIV-3. To do so, slide the index finger between the big toe and second toe, until you reach a cavity right before the intersection of the metatarsals (the bones of the feet). Point LIV-3 is easier to locate when the index finger hooks around the metatarsal of the big toe. Do not confuse point LIV-3 with points LIV-1 and LIV-2 situated along the big toe (*illustration 6.4*).
2. **During rushes**, apply firm and painful pressure to point LIV-3.

Beneficial Effects:

Relieves stress and clears the mind.

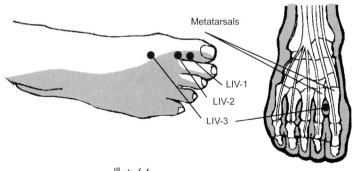

Illustr. 6.4

Stimulating the spleen, or point SP-6-Sanyinjiao

SP-6 is well-known in Chinese medicine and scientific literature for its pain-reducing effect. It is easy to find and is generally very painful.

1. Before applying painful pressure, you must find point SP-6. To do so:

   - Find the malleolus of the ankle (on the inside of the leg).
   - Find the central and protruding point of the malleolus.
   - Place the *woman's* four fingers horizontally, starting at the protruding point of the malleolus. Point SP-6 is on the inner side of the leg and against the bone of the tibia (*illustration 6.5*).

2. **During rushes**, apply firm and painful pressure to this point.

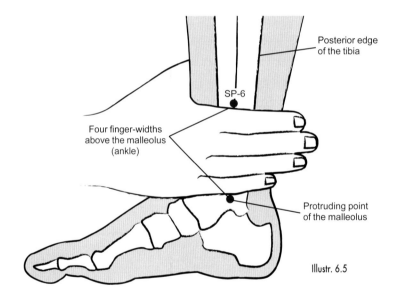

Posterior edge of the tibia

SP-6

Four finger-widths above the malleolus (ankle)

Protruding point of the malleolus

Illustr. 6.5

Beneficial Effects:
- Works with the other acupuncture reflex zones to help induce and establish labor.
- Helps dilate the cervix efficiently.
- Calms the mind and the body.
- Reduces pain[174].

Stimulating the heart, or point H-7-Shenmen

Point H-7 is sometimes difficult to locate, since it does not always create a distinct numb sensation. To help you find this point, locate the pisiform bone and the tendon. The pisiform bone is a small knobbly, pea-shaped bone, embedded in a tendon, that is found in the wrist. Start with the left hand, as in illustration 6.6.

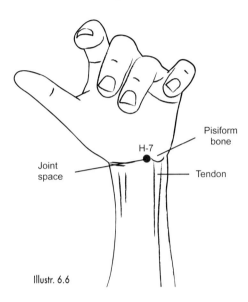

Pisiform bone

H-7

Joint space

Tendon

Illustr. 6.6

Before applying painful pressure, you must find point H-7. To do so:

1. Start with the left hand, lightly flex the fist to make the tendon appear on the little finger side.
2. Find the pisiform bone in the wrist, which is located at the end of the tendon. Point H-7 is situated on the inner edge of the pisiform bone.
3. **During rushes**, apply firm and painful pressure.

Beneficial Effects:
Calms the mind and the body.

PRACTICAL EXERCISE: RECEIVING A MASSAGE
When you experience fatigue and tension in the lower body, ask for a gentle massage of the sacrum, the hips, and of the buttock muscles.

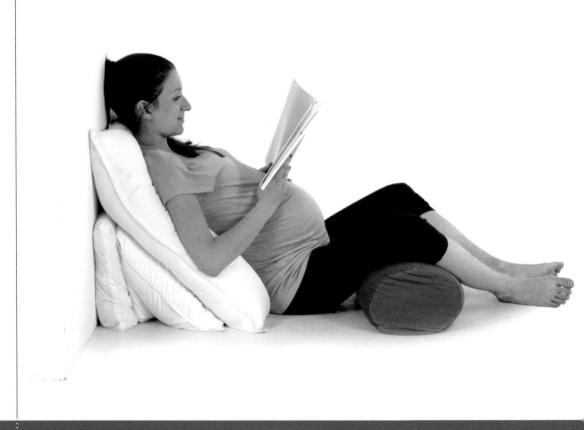

Chapter 7

RELAXATION

Stress can have a positive and stimulating effect, but if it is not frequently released, it can exhaust you and severely reduce your quality of life.

Rest and relaxation are important parts of health at any time. During pregnancy and birth, they are particularly important. They prevent fatigue, ensure physical and mental well-being, neutralize body tensions and strong sensations at the time of birth, and prepare you for the practice of mental imagery.

Summary of Chapter 7: Relaxation

OBJECTIVE	METHOD
◆ Neutralize stress, fatigue and discomfort	◆ Practice relaxation
◆ Prepare for mental imagery (chapter 8)	◆ Practice relaxation
◆ Neutralize the fear-tension-pain cycle ◆ Promote a calm and confident attitude ◆ Let go of sensations that come and go	◆ Practice relaxation

During birth, the role of the companion is to remind the woman to relax and to abandon herself to the strong sensations.

The role of the woman is to relax and stay calm, and to neutralize the sources of tension.

NEUTRALIZING FEAR THROUGH RELAXATION

In the 1930s, the British obstetrician Dr. Grantly Dick-Read was a fervent advocate for natural birth. Over the course of his practice, he observed that fear and anxiety create tensions that, in turn, accentuate pain. This is the fear-tension-pain cycle[175]. You can alleviate the effects of this vicious cycle by preparing yourself mentally and by practicing techniques for modulating strong sensations. By mental repetition of positive affirmations (e.g. "I am doing well and I am calm"), you will be able to better manage your potentially painful sensations. You will be able to better adapt to the unknowns of birth.

Relaxation plays a key role in the experience of birth. Relaxed, the body revitalizes itself and produces a state of well-being throughout your whole body. In addition, using mental and thought control of the central nervous system (third mechanism), relaxation can help you view rushes as essential to the process of labor. At birth, relaxation induced by breathing is used during rushes to relax the jaw, the abdominal muscles, the adductors (inner thigh muscles) and the muscles of the perineum. Learning relaxation with the help of an audio recording will help you to become familiar with the basics of active and passive relaxation methods. The more you practice, the better the results will be. Remember that the sensations come and go. *After night comes day*.

This chapter proposes methods and tips to teach you to relax. Here are some suggestions to apply, no matter the place or time you choose to relax.

- Practice relaxation under dimmed lighting, away from distracting noises, in loose clothing, at a comfortable temperature, to better relax your muscles.
- Create your physical relaxation by choosing the approach that works best for you. If you are already good at an effective relaxation method, use that one.
- Plan for one period of relaxation per day.
- If you work on a schedule, make the most out of your down-time (breaks and lunch time). Also take time to relax between work and any other obligation.
- Learn to relax over the course of pregnancy and you will be able to do so during the birth.

Tension can cause discomfort and a slowing down of labor's progress. Rest and relaxation reduce fatigue and help you to respond to the demands of birth.

SOME RELAXATION POSTURES

You can relax in each of the postures described in the following paragraphs. Practice relaxation whenever you are resting.

Lying on Your Back

This posture is particularly comfortable at the beginning of pregnancy, but may cause problems if used later on, due to the weight of the baby on the vena cava (vein situated along your back that carries blood to your heart) and the lower back.

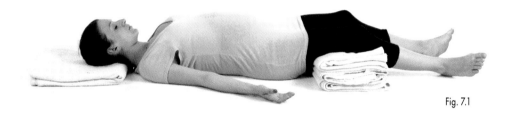

Fig. 7.1

1. Place a semi-rigid support under the knees. Place a folded blanket under your head (the forehead is slightly sloping down toward the chest).
2. Lie on your back by placing your hands on the floor to one side and using your thighs to roll onto your side.
3. Widen your buttocks by grabbing the flesh under your sit bones and gently stretching them to the sides so that your lower back is well-supported on the floor.
4. Release your legs and let your feet fall outward. To open the chest, roll the shoulders back and down toward the waist
5. Extend your arms to your sides and turn your palms upward facing the ceiling. Arms are at a 45 degree angle from the body.
6. Make sure the head is centered and in line with the spine.
7. Pay attention to the symmetry of your body. Allow your upper eyelids to lower onto the bottom ones, relax your eyes in their sockets and release all tension accumulated around the eyes, temples, and lips.

Lying on the Side of Your Belly

This position is restful during the last phase of pregnancy, and during labor.

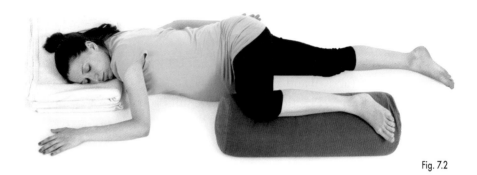

Fig. 7.2

- Lie on the side of your belly, by turning slightly to your preferred side. Note, however, that lying on your left side will promote better blood circulation.
- Extend the arm behind you. Bend it slightly.
- Put your head and part of your chest on the floor.
- To rest your back and abdomen, bend your front leg slightly by resting it on a support (*figure 7.2*).

Lying on Your Side

Just like the previous position, this one is relaxing during the last phase of pregnancy, and during labor.

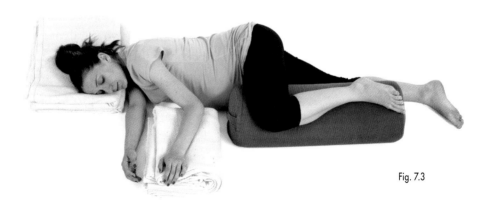

Fig. 7.3

TRUSTING BIRTH WITH THE BONAPACE METHOD

- Lie on your preferred side. Occasionally switch sides.
- Rest your head on a support.
- Gently bend the front leg by putting it on a support (*figure 7.3*).
- Extend one arm in front of you. Rest the other arm on a support in front of you.

RELAXATION METHODS

Researchers have devised two simple methods for learning relaxation: progressive muscular relaxation[176] (active) and autogenous relaxation[177] (passive). Below, I provide practical examples of both. Practice the one that suits you best, or combine the two. What is important is to know that only daily practice will bring you to mastery of relaxation. At the beginning, you may have the impression that you are wasting your time; your thoughts may be agitated and you will feel impatient. Once your body becomes familiar with complete relaxation, which is very different from what we consider a relaxed state, it will start asking for this more often. From then on, the simple act of getting into the relaxation posture will be enough to cause rapid relaxation of the whole body.

PRACTICAL EXERCISE: ACTIVE AND PASSIVE METHODS

Since practice is the best way to learn relaxation, in the following paragraphs I will introduce two daily exercises.

Progressive Muscular Relaxation (Active)

Progressive muscular relaxation is a method that suits people who have difficulty concentrating. It focuses on the difference between tension and relaxation.

1. Get into the relaxation posture of your choice (*figures 7.1, 7.2 or 7.3*).
2. Close your eyes and pay attention to your breathing for a few moments.
3. Follow this with the breathing exercise from chapter 4 (two spirals of 12 breaths).
4. Progressive muscular relaxation is composed of three steps: Flex a muscle as tightly as you can. Observe the tension you feel. Relax the muscle and pay attention to the difference between the two sensations: flexed muscle and relaxed muscle.
5. Start by flexing your feet. Lift the heels off the floor and flex the toes toward your knees. Note the sensation that this movement creates: the muscles are

taut and stiff, and the feet tremble a bit. Feel the tension in your feet. Maintain this flexing for a few seconds. While you are flexing your feet, relax all other parts of your body.

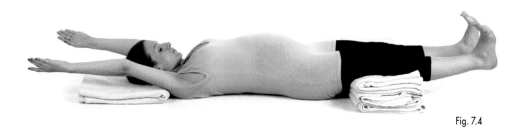

Fig. 7.4

6. Release the tension in your feet. Relax them. The tension disappears. Note how much heavier the feet feel than when they were flexed. They have lost their tension.
7. Notice the difference in sensation between flexed and relaxed feet. Do your feet feel prickly, or are they hot? Did the tension you felt when your foot was flexed disappear as soon as you released your foot?
8. Continue by creating tension in each large group of muscles. Progress from the feet towards the head, or from the head to the feet, by relaxing the muscles in the legs, abdomen, pelvis, back, arms, hands, and face. The basic technique does not change: flex the muscle, release the tension, and note the difference.
9. Another variation is to contract all muscles at the same time, release the tension, then note the difference (*figure 7.4*).

Working on all the major muscle groups only takes a few minutes. This exercise can be practiced sitting or lying down; try it in a calm and relaxed atmosphere, wearing loose clothing.

The following exercise will help you to feel the results of passive relaxation. This practice prepares you to induce relaxation for the birth.

Autogenous Relaxation (Passive)

Autogenous relaxation puts the mind before the body. By simple suggestion, you condition your body by telling it how it should feel. You will receive a relaxation response each time that you feel stressed or tense.

1. Take up a relaxation posture (*figures 7.1, 7.2 or 7.3*).
2. Close your eyes and pay attention to your breathing for a few moments.
3. Follow this with the breathing exercise from chapter 4 (two spirals of 12 breaths).
4. Repeat soothing phrases, such as "I am calm", "I am well", etc.
5. Concentrate on the different parts of your body. Start at the feet and continue all the way to the head, or vice versa. Mentally repeat that the part of the body that you wish to relax is warm and heavy, for example: "my right hand is warm and heavy. It is warmer and heavier." Repeat each affirmation 3 times. Do the same thing while concentrating on your left hand, left leg, etc, until you are completely relaxed.
6. To finish the exercise, breathe deeply and stretch.
7. Open your eyes, exhale gently and observe how you feel.
8. Note down in your notebook what you've experienced.

This technique works well for those who can concentrate easily. Its practice requires time, and most importantly, determination. Begin by practicing twice a day, 10 minutes each time. After four to eight weeks, you will reach a satisfying level of relaxation in only 5 minutes. As you progress, you will see that it becomes easier and easier to relax at will. By perfecting these techniques, you will be able to relax anywhere, anytime.

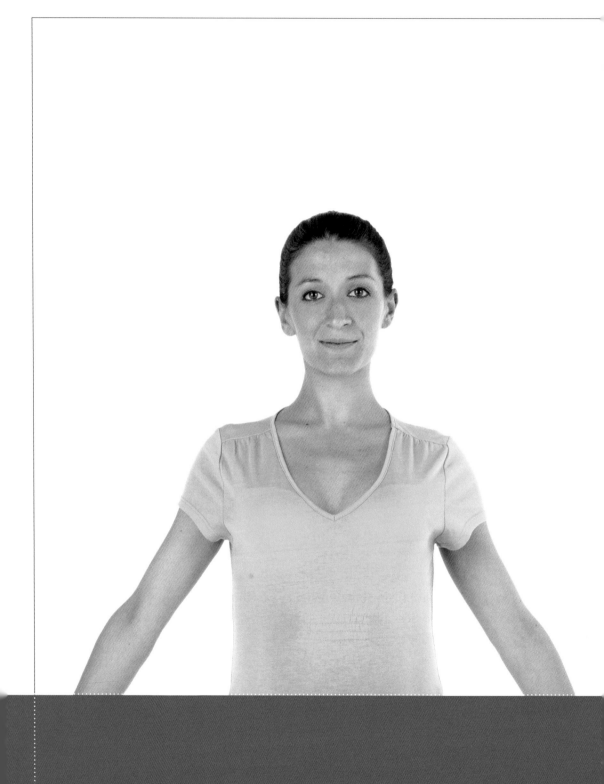

Chapitre 8

PSYCHOLOGICAL PREPARATION

Pyschological preparation is part of controlling the central nervous system through your thoughts and mind. It is one of the methods associated with the third mechanism for modulating (or altering) the strong sensations of birth. As you already know, this mechanism is activated during labor and birth by the continuous support of a loving person, by conscious breathing, relaxation, mental imagery, and, in a more comprehensive sense, cognition.

Cognition enables us to give personal significance to such an event as labor and birth (e.g. "Birth is natural; women have been doing it since the dawn of time"). Through cognition, we also perceive the security of the event (e.g. "Giving birth is risky; many complications can arise"). Cognition is also responsible for the manner in which we perceive our own capabilities (e.g. "I have within me all the internal mechanisms and resources necessary to give birth" or "Others are more competent than I am").

Throughout this book, we have demonstrated how your body is an extraordinary resource in the growing and birthing of your child. Through careful reading of the different chapters, you have been able to restructure your thoughts in such a way so as to understand that you possess all that is needed to give birth; this is positive cognition. You have learned that certain yoga poses will allow you to develop the strength and flexibility needed to carry and bring your child into the world. You have also observed that a strong hormonal system, already present in your body, is designed to help you birth your baby with ease, pleasure and safety.

You also understand that the mechanisms that allow for the modification of signals sent to your brain allow you to modulate (or alter) strong sensations that are associated with rushes. Finally, you have discovered that conscious breathing, making sounds, and the capacity to welcome strong emotions linked to labor are also resources at your disposal. These are all resources that allow you to give birth in a satisfying manner.

Research[178] has shown that certain techniques related to this third mechanism, control of the nervous system by thought, reduce the frequency of obstetrical interventions while simultaneously improving infant health and maternal satisfaction. From this, we can presume that if the mother is psychologically prepared for pregnancy and birth, she will experience less fear and anxiety. This zen state (i.e. less fear and anxiety) creates an environment that is favorable to birth.

In the following paragraphs, you will be introduced to three psychological preparation techniques to help you create your own zen state during pregnancy and birth:

- Practicing positive attitude and gratefulness;
- Emotional Freedom Technique (EFT);
- Mental imagery.

This chapter will help you to integrate a zen attitude into your daily life.

Summary of Chapter 8: Psychological Preparation

OBJECTIVE	METHOD
• Adopt a zen state during pregnancy and birth • Manage strong sensations during the birth	• Practice positive attitude and gratitude to reduce anxiety and stress • Practice the Emotional Freedom Technique (EFT) in order to recognize and accept negative emotions, to then transform them into positive emotions • Direct your attention using mental imagery
• Condition positive messages in relation to the steps that inspire a certain apprehension	• Practice positive attitude and gratitude • Watch films or discuss with an inspiring resource person
• Recognize negative emotions	• Practice the Emotional Freedom Technique to free your emotions
• Develop a healthy vision of birth, in order to prevent disappointment	• Formulate realistic goals related to labor and birth (avoid rigid models that don't leave room for the unexpected) • Visualize multiple scenarios founded on an attitude of calm and confidence

If they want to prepare themselves psychologically for birth, the mother and her partner need to experiment with different psychological techniques in order to be able to create their own zen zone during pregnancy and birth. Both must also create the conditions for a satisfying and secure birth, while knowing to surrender to the unknown.

POSITIVISM AND GRATITUDE

Our thoughts influence our emotions, and our emotions influence our body. A positive attitude requires you to see what is going well, rather than what is not going well. It requires you to recognize what is beautiful and good in each situation. Thoughts created in this way stimulate the secretion of endorphins (hormone of pleasure, transcendence, relief). They also stimulate the release of oxytocin, the hormone of love that generates well-being and improves health. We can prove these with a basic experiment: Simply think of someone you adore. Think of their presence, their smile, their embrace, your conversation with them. Your heart opens and you feel relaxed and happy. On the other hand, think of a conflict you have gone through. Think of the words that triggered the conflict. As you ponder these thoughts, notice your body tensing up.

Repetition of positive affirmations and the expression of gratitude are examples of tools that can help you to maintain a positive perspective, in order to create your own space of well-being.

Positive Affirmations

Here are some examples of affirmations to repeat multiple times per day, out loud (or mentally), during pregnancy and birth.

- I have what it takes to grow my baby and give birth.
- My body and my baby know how to work together.
- Giving birth is safe for my baby and for me.

Think of your own personal affirmations that will focus your attention on a pleasant pregnancy and satisfying birth. Formulate your affirmations in the present tense, in the indicative mode ("I am…", "I feel…", "I see myself…"), rather than in the conditional mode ("I would like…", "I would feel…", "I would see myself") and give them a positive form ("I am calm" rather than "I am not stressed").

Expressing Gratitude

To help you cultivate positive sensations, practice the following exercise regularly, for 15 to 20 minutes. It will allow you to combine multiple other tools presented in this book. This exercise is about gratitude, a virtue that opens the heart and leads straight to the zen state.

1. Get into a comfortable relaxation position.
2. Chant the sound HU (pronounced HUE) out loud, to develop your breathing capacity and to relax your perineal and respiratory diaphragms. You can also chant it quietly or mentally.
3. While you chant, bring your attention to the zone between your eyebrows, a few centimeters inside your skull, without straining your eyes.
4. Imagine a screen on which you can see the positive and pleasant aspects of your day[179]. Start with the present moment and go back all the way to when you woke up in the morning.
5. Remember each little sensation, situation, emotion or thought that was pleasant to you: a smile, food that you ate, a delightful impression, warmth on your body, your baby's movement, an embrace, etc.
6. Feel the warm, calm, soothing effect oxytocin brings to your body.

EMOTIONAL FREEDOM FOR STRESS REDUCTION

The Emotional Freedom Technique (EFT)[180, 181] requires us to recognize negative emotions that we experience, in order to objectify and question them, so that we can find a more optimal mindset – the zen state. It is important to recognize your negative emotions and to vent them. This way, what is expressed does not leave traces of tension, pain, and eventually illness and disease in the body.

The Emotional Freedom Technique is a form of self-treatment. Its aim is to reduce stress using energy circuits in the body, while working on specific emotions. In this way, EFT combines two therapeutic approaches: acupuncture (Chinese energy medicine) and the conventional psychotherapy approach that aims to restructure thought by the use of words and images.

This technique was developed with an understanding that intense negative emotions or traumatic events put your body in a state of alert, by activating your stress response system. The release of stress hormones (adrenaline and cortisol, among others) prepares your body to fight, flee or freeze. Even when the situation is only of minor importance (being late for an appointment, too much work, disorganized environment, noise, etc), your hormones activate a stress response. If it is not frequently released, stress fatigues the body and mind.

The goal of this technique is to stop the activation of the stress response system by negative emotions, and to reprogram the mind so that it reacts differently. During birth, a reduction in stress will have multiple benefits. Namely, it will allow you to be in a state where your natural hormones reach an optimal flow, which makes labor easy, efficient and safe.

The technique consists of eight simple steps that you can put into practice each time you feel an intense negative feeling, or whenever you relive a painful memory. Self-treatment with EFT takes only a few minutes, and can be practiced at any time, with the goal of helping you regain your zen state[182].

1. Define the statement of importance that you want to tackle (the situation that is bothering you) and write a reminder phrase, for example: "Birth. I am very afraid of this event."
2. Evaluate the intensity of your feelings related to that statement on a scale of 0 to 10, 0 being the least intense, and 10 being the most intense.
3. Create the set up statement that begins with "Even though…"; add the emotion you experienced (present or past); add the situation that is bothering you (the context); and add the desired outcome (the result) that you choose. For example: "Even though I feel stressed and am afraid (emotions) of giving birth (context), I choose to love and accept myself and to trust my body (the desired result)."

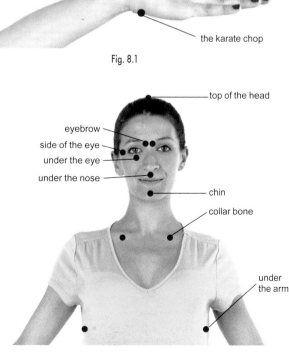

Fig. 8.1

the karate chop

top of the head
eyebrow
side of the eye
under the eye
under the nose
chin
collar bone
under the arm

Fig. 8.2

4. Repeat the set up statement three times while using all the fingers of

one hand to tap the "karate chop" point located on the side of the opposite hand (*figure 8.1*).

5. Repeat the statement of importance as you repeatedly tap on each of the acupuncture reflex points (remember to complete the statement before moving on to the next point). Tap one side of your face or body at a time, or both simultaneously (*figure 8.2*). As you progress, you will describe in a more precise and detailed way the context and the feelings that you experience. If other emotions surface, describe them. Continue until the intense emotions dissipate. For example: "Birth. I am very afraid of this event." If you are experiencing difficulty in finding the proper words, imagine yourself having a conversation with your best friend.

    ◆ **Between the eyebrows:** "Birth. I am very afraid of this event."
    ◆ **Side of the eye:** "Giving birth is difficult and risky."
    ◆ **Under the eye:** "I am afraid for my health."
    ◆ **Under the nose:** "I am afraid for the health of my baby, whom I love."
    ◆ **Chin:** "I do not feel safe."
    ◆ **Collar bone:** "I do not want to suffer."
    ◆ **Under the arm:** "I don't have what it takes to give birth naturally."
    ◆ **Top of the head:** "In the past, women were stronger and more robust."
    ◆ **Between the eyebrows:** "They let themselves be guided by their instinct."
    ◆ **Side of the eye:** "Giving birth was simple, efficient and safe."
    ◆ **Under the eye:** "Women always knew how to give birth."
    ◆ **Under the nose:** "They trusted their bodies, because they didn't have a choice."
    ◆ **Chin:** "They had to rely on their internal mechanisms and resources."
    ◆ **Collar bone:** "They relied on memories encoded in their DNA."
    ◆ **Under the arm:** "They tolerated pain."
    ◆ **Top of the head:** "These women knew, but I don't."

6. Migrate toward positive affirmations by exploring which of your negative ideas are erroneous (e.g. "I don't have what it takes to give birth"), by looking to your real needs (e.g. "I need to feel safe" or "I need to feel respected") and by identifying the paths that will lead you to the outcome that you chose in your set up statement (i.e. "Even though, …") Continue the positive, exploratory affirmations while continuing to tap the acupuncture reflex points.

- Between the eyebrows: "Is it possible that my generation doesn't know how to give birth?"
- Side of the eye: "Is it possible that the internal mechanisms and resources for getting through birth no longer exist?"
- Under the eye: "What can I do to give birth like my ancestors?"
- Under the nose: "How can I transform my fears into power?"
- Chin: "I have what it takes to give birth."
- Collar bone: "I have the capabilities needed to give birth."
- Under the arms: "Giving birth is natural."
- Top of the head: "My baby and I are laboring together. We will know what to do."

7. Exhale completely and breathe deeply.
8. Evaluate the intensity of your feelings on the scale from 0 to 10, and compare your results to your initial score.

Why negative affirmations? When one is inhabited by fears, limiting beliefs or parasitic thoughts, an inner dialogue occurs. This discussion, whether inward or out loud, is perceived by the body as a stress. The repetition of negative thoughts further compounds the problem. The stimulation of acupuncture reflex points at the same time as the repetition of negative affirmations allows these emotions to be vented and to rewire the brain to create new associations to those thoughts.

Sometimes, the outcome of your tapping session will be to make a concrete gesture (e.g. affirming your need), while other situations will require surrender or letting go (i.e. trusting, and entering a zen state). The key to success lies in regular practice. If needed, do not hesitate to contact an EFT professional to guide you in the use of this technique.

The next time you have an intense negative emotion or stress, put the different steps of the Emotional Freedom Technique into practice.

MENTAL IMAGERY

Just like the other two techniques suggested in this chapter, the goal of utilizing mental imagery is to help you find out what you need in order to feel good and to create your own zen zone. It is a technique that anyone can use, at any time in their life. However, it is not always used consciously, or in a positive manner.

When you pack your bags for a trip, you imagine the place you are going, the weather and the activities that you will engage in. You want to include clothing in your luggage that will be appropriate for the trip. You will choose what is useful and leave what is not. Ultimately, you want to take what is needed for each activity, taking into account the conditions that will exist when you get there. Projecting an image of yourself into the future in order to figure out what clothing you will need is basically the same as practicing mental imagery.

Mental imagery works in two different ways:

- It helps you to consciously direct your attention.
- It allows you to access your inner worlds.

The first step in practicing mental imagery is to choose a situation or event for which you wish to prepare yourself (e.g. birth). The exercise could be about a situation in general (for example: the whole birth, from start to finish), or about a very specific part of a situation (e.g. the beginning of labor, relaxing the perineum, or bearing down).

When you practice mental imagery, you consciously direct your attention toward that which you want to work on. To keep your attention on the object of your imagery, you visualize details: the visual aspect of the place (the room, the furniture, the people around you, the light), the sensations (heat, calm, well-being, confidence, love, peace), the scents and the gestures or actions of yourself and those around you (who does what, and how).

You imagine the scenario in a positive manner. You avoid focusing on negative scenarios by giving them too many details. Rather, you repeat: "No matter what situation I face, I choose to stay calm and confident. I know what to do in the face of all unknowns."

Practicing will develop your capacity to become aware of your thoughts and to redirect them as needed. In this way, if you are given bad news, you won't panic by thinking about all the possible negative consequences associated with this event. You will concentrate on the present moment, with the information you have available. You direct your thoughts to what you know and to realistic and optimistic scenarios. This prevents over-dramatization, which increases stress even more.

For example, at your 36-week appointment, you learn that your baby is breech. Do not let your emotions and irrational thoughts take over by imagining all of the stages that could occur between the present and the birth. Rather, pay attention to what you know: the baby is in breech position. Recognize the emotions that you are feeling (for example, fear and anxiety). Use the Emotional Freedom Technique to vent the emotions and to migrate toward a plan of action. Stay focused on what you *can* do and on what *belongs* to you. For example, you *can* practice positions for turning a baby, request consultation with an acupuncturist or an osteopath, etc. Practicing mental imagery will help you to follow and focus your train of thought.

PRACTICAL EXERCISE: YOUR BIRTH SCENARIO

To help you to use mental imagery, here is a birth scenario that you can modify and personalize as you see fit. The key words are calm and confidence.

1. Get into a comfortable relaxation position.
2. Chant the sound HU (pronounced HUE)[183] out loud, to develop your breathing capacity and to relax your perineal and respiratory diaphragms. You can also chant it quietly or mentally.
3. As you chant, bring your attention to the zone between your eyebrows, a few centimeters inside your skull, without straining your eyes.
4. Imagine a screen on which you can see the scenario described below.
5. At the end of the exercise, note what you saw and felt. Repeat the exercise by imagining the whole scenario or specific parts.

My partner and I are at home, on a Sunday, and all is calm. My pregnancy has reached full term, and we feel good. I have had rushes for two days. I appreciate them, since they are telling me that my body knows what to do. I accept them with gratitude, and let them come and go. I am calm and confident.

I take the time to savor these last moments of my pregnancy. I go for a stroll with my partner. I feel zen, really in my zone. I have confidence that I have what it takes to bring my child into the world. I don't have a fixed idea about how it has to happen. I'm just very confident that I'll know what to do. I feel safe. I am protected and calm.

My partner is excited. He is so eager to see the baby and to put into practice what he knows. He asks me questions and watches me. I reassure him by telling him that I will know what to do when the time comes. I invite him to remain in this zen state with me and to trust birth.

Time passes and doesn't matter. I'm observing my sensations and living the present moment. The sensations grow stronger, and I welcome them. I thank my body and its wisdom for this labor which continues to make its way, one rush at a time. I am calm and feel love for this baby and for my partner. Each rush brings me closer to my baby, whom I so dearly wish to hold in my arms. I breathe her scent, smallness, delicateness and gentleness. She is also eager to be born. Together, we know what to do. I feel my hormones circulating in both of us. We are calm, confident and safe.

The rushes through my belly are more persistent, and demand more and more of my attention. I stop talking, exhale completely, relax my mouth and buttocks and let the sensations appear and disappear. My partner's embrace, skin to skin contact, and deep kisses help me to relax. I feel the increases in oxytocin and love, and the intensification of my rushes. I am thankful and calm. I give thanks to my body, which knows what to do.

It is now clear that I am in active labor, because my rushes are becoming more intense, closer together, and longer. They really require my full attention. That is fine with me, because I know that these strong rushes are allowing my cervix to ripen and soften, to efface and thin, and to dilate and open. My partner is calm and presses my trigger points during rushes. I feel an increase in endorphins, which cradles me and allows me to take some distance from my intense sensations. I am well, and calm.

(Adjust the scenario according to the place where you will give birth. If you plan to give birth at home, with midwives attending, imagine that you telephone them and that they come to meet you. If you plan to give birth at a birthing center or hospital, notify the staff by telephone of the progression of your labor, and of your imminent arrival. Get comfortable in your room, in the place where you will labor.)

The rushes continue. I move, I make sounds, I breathe and I am calm. I trust my body, my baby, my partner, and all those who accompany me on this journey. I welcome each emotion as it presents itself. I continue to eat and hydrate myself, according to how I feel. I am patient, patient, and still patient. Everyone around me is so devoted and attentive. I thank them inwardly.

I don't know how long I've been there, nor how many centimeters dilated I am. These factors are not important for me. I stay in the present and live one rush at a time. I keep all my attention on my breathing, and exhale completely, chanting HU (pronounced HUE). I am confident. I think of my baby, who is thriving on my endorphins. She is also being guided and kept company. We're waiting ... she's coming. Thank you baby!

The sensations are strong. My goodness, am I going to get through this? What happens if...? It's too much, I'm tearing and breaking inside! Is something wrong? That's not possible. I feel submerged, overwhelmed...

I welcome my sensations, my imperfections, since it's my body who is in charge. The stress hormones are working to facilitate delivery. Ok, hang in there! I continue.

TRUSTING BIRTH WITH THE BONAPACE METHOD

Tapping calms me. Other women have done this, thousands of generations before me. I know what to do. I let myself be. I welcome my sensations.

My attitude changes; I sense this strength, the strength of the tigress, the wolf, the lioness, all the females of the world. It is this indomitable strength that brings my baby into the world. I can feel the baby's head with my hands at my vulva. She is there, so close. She wants to be born, so that we can finally be together. I observe my body which pushes the child toward the light of day. I feel her head and body making their way. She is there, finally, whole and hot on my body, skin to skin. We look at each other, eye to eye, and I feel myself falling even more in love with her. She is awake, alert, and we are both still swimming in a hormonal sea of endorphins, oxytocin, and prolactin. It is the beginning of our co-dependence, which will be good for both of us. She touches me, caresses me, and suckles my breast. I feel the oxytocin rising in me. This is love, unconditional and limitless. Welcome, my baby!

The rushes continue, to birth the baby's placenta, the organ that allowed her to develop. I give thanks to life, to the wisdom of my body, to my baby, my partner, and all who are with me on this wonderful journey.

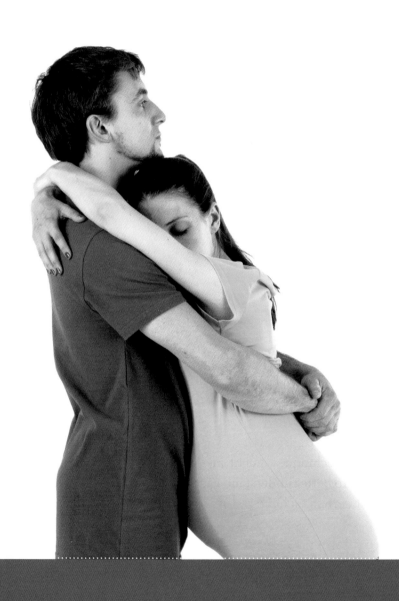

BY WAY OF CONCLUSION

Pregnancy and birth are a step that prepare you for your long-term commitment to your child. No matter what happens during birth, be confident and calm. These two qualities will allow you to remain centered and adapt to the unknown as it unfolds.

During this period, your relationship with your partner will experience a transition, since the birth of the family creates changes and necessitates adaptation. Take care of your relationship: it is the basis of your family. Get in the habit of making time for the two of you. For example, enjoy time alone and take a few days off every once in a while to recharge and rekindle the love between you two. Take every chance to fully live the experience of being parents.

After the birth of your child, it is possible that you will experience difficulties adapting to the many changes that family life demands. Don't hesitate to ask for help. You will not be the first to sometimes feel overwhelmed and isolated. Ask family members and people in your entourage and community. These people can help you over the course of this transition.

Through the techniques taught in this book, you will certainly have discovered how it is possible to better understand each other and support each other. You will have a preference for certain techniques (breathing, exercises, massage, relaxation, tapping and mental imagery). No matter which ones you choose, what is important is that you are able to work together to find comfort in difficult moments. Don't forget that the skills you acquired during pregnancy and birth are now part of you, part of your arsenal of resources, and that they will follow you into the next stages of your life.

I wish you many wonderful moments with your child!

Appendix 1

BIRTH TRAVEL BAGS AND BABY SUPPLIES CHECKLIST

Mother's Bag

Prepare your bag at least 4 weeks before your due date.

- Toothbrush and toothpaste
- Hairbrush and comb
- Deodorant
- Soap
- Breast pads
- Sanitary pads
- Underwear (2)
- Bras (2)
- Light pyjamas that open in front, for breastfeeding
- Bathrobe
- Socks (2 pairs)
- Slippers
- Pencil or pen
- Clothes for leaving the hospital (size: about 4 months pregnant)
- Health Insurance Card
- Hospital card (if applicable)
- Insurance/hospitalization documents
- Social Security number

Baby's Bag

- Onesie
- Pyjamas
- Hat
- Sweater
- In winter, prepare a wool outfit and a winter outfit
- Small swaddling blanket
- Bigger blanket to protect against wind, even in summer
- Car seat
- Diapers

Partner's Bag

Labor can last more than 24 hours. Make sure you have everything for your comfort, and the mother's, as well as food.

- Socks (2 pairs)
- Light, short-sleeved t-shirts (2)
- Lavender, jasmine or sage essential oil (must be a type that the mother likes)
- Massage oil or cream

- Yoga mat
- Wooden massage tools
- Ice pack
- Hot water bottle
- 'Magic bag' (heatable)
- Rebozo (large sheet or scarf)
- Marker to identify acupuncture zones
- Ball for moving in labor
- Flameless candles to create atmospheric lighting
- Easily digestible foods: cooked root vegetables (carrots, beets, parsnips, turnips), toast, fruit, nuts, honey, broth, herbal teas (chamomile or fennel for nausea), coconut water, energy drinks rich in electrolytes. Prepare hot meals that do not have strong odors that could cause nausea.
- Chewing gum and mouthwash for fresh breath

- Size 6 months socks (2 or 3 pairs)
- Warm blanket, preferably wool
- Diaper bag
- Baby formula, if baby is not breastfed

Toiletries
- Baby bathtub (optional)
- Small bath towels (4)
- Cotton swabs
- Round cotton pads
- Rubbing alcohol
- Rectal thermometer
- Small, round-ended scissors
- Gentle (hypoallergenic) soap
- Unscented oil

Furniture
- Safe crib with firm mattress
- Changing table (optional)

Baby's Room
Clothing
- Short-sleeved cotton onesies (6)
- Size 0-3 months pyjamas (1 or 2)
- Size 3-6 months pyjamas (4 to 6)
- Cloth diapers (2 or 3 dozen)
- Bags of disposable diapers (2 or 3)
- Small flannel blankets (6)
- Bib
- Sheets/mattress covers (3)
- Sweater
- Hat

TRUSTING BIRTH WITH THE BONAPACE METHOD

RECIPES

Fortifying Broth for Mother

This broth is excellent for calming and soothing the nervous system[184]. Use organic ingredients if possible.

2 cups of sweet potato, cubed
1 cup of leek, cut into sections
1 cup of Swiss chard (in the same family as beets), cut into strips
1 cup of green beans, chopped
1 cup of carrot with leaves, chopped
1 cup of kale, chopped
1 yellow onion with skin, chopped
6 sprigs of parsley, roughly chopped
2 or 3 whole garlic cloves
1/4 cup seaweed (kombu, dulse, nori or wakame)
5 cm piece of fresh ginger, cut into strips

Wash and cut the vegetables. Keep the skin if the vegetable is organic and has been washed carefully. Place all ingredients in a large pot and cover with water. Simmer gently for 3 to 5 hours. Filter and add sea salt or fleur de sel, or curry powder.

Raspberry Leaf Infusion

Raspberry leaves (wild or cultivated) are made into an infusion to soothe diarrhea and nausea. The infusion works as a tonic on the uterus and the muscles of the digestive system, while preventing spasms. It is used during painful and abundant menstruation or to facilitate birth[185].

1. Infuse approximately 50 fresh raspberry leaves or 4 tsp dried leaves in a liter of boiling water. Let sit for 10 minutes.
2. Prepare ice chips for labor made with hibiscus flower infusion or raspberry leaves.

Lemon Energy Drink

This drink is rich in vitamins and minerals. It soothes nausea and gives energy.

4 cups of water or coconut water
1/3 cup unpasteurized honey (in this form, it retains the most enzymes and vitamins)
1/4 to 1/2 tsp sea salt or fleur de sel (avoid commercial table salt, as it contains anti-caking agents and stabilizers)
1 tbsp chia seeds (rich in protein, fiber, magnesium and calcium)
juice of 2 or 3 fresh lemons

Into a closed 1 liter container, pour 1/2 cup lukewarm water, then add the honey, salt and chia seeds. Mix to dissolve, and add the rest of the water and lemon juice. It is normal for chia seeds to become glutinous after being soaked in water.

Appendix 3

MOTHERBABY RIGHTS

From www.imbci.org

1. You and your baby have the right to be treated with respect and dignity.
2. You have the right to be involved in and fully informed about care for yourself and your baby.
3. You have the right to be communicated with in a language and in terminology that you understand.
4. You have the right to informed consent and to informed refusal for any treatment, procedure or other aspect of care for yourself and your baby.
5. You and your baby have the right to receive care that enhances and optimizes the normal processes of pregnancy, birth and postpartum under a model known as the midwifery (or mother-baby) model of care.
6. You and your baby have the right to receive continuous support during labor and birth from those you choose.
7. You have the right to be offered drug-free comfort and pain-relief measures during labor and to have the benefits of these measures and the means of their use explained to you and to your companions.
8. You and your baby have the right to receive care consisting of evidence-based practices proven to be beneficial in supporting the normal physiology of labor, birth and postpartum.
9. You and your baby have the right to receive care that seeks to avoid potentially harmful procedures and practices.
10. You have the right to receive education concerning a healthy environment and disease prevention.
11. You have the right to receive education regarding responsible sexuality, family planning and women's reproductive rights, as well as access to family planning options.

12. You have the right to receive supportive prenatal, intrapartum, postpartum and newborn care that addresses your physical and emotional health within the context of family relationships and your community environment.

13. You and your baby have the right to evidenced-based emergency treatment for life-threatening complications.

14. You and your baby have the right to be cared for by a small number of care providers who collaborate across disciplinary, cultural and institutional boundaries and who provide consultations and facilitate transfers of care when necessary to appropriate institutions and specialists.

15. You have the right to be made aware of and to be shown how to access available community services for yourself and your baby.

16. You and your baby have the right to be cared for by practitioners with knowledge of and the skills to support breastfeeding.

17. You have the right to be educated concerning the benefits and the management of breastfeeding and to be shown how to breastfeed and how to maintain lactation, even if you and your baby must be separated for medical reasons.

18. You and your baby have the right to initiate breastfeeding within the first 30 minutes after birth, to remain together skin-to-skin for at least the first hour, to stay together 24 hours a day and to breastfeed on demand.

19. Your baby has the right to be given no artificial teats or pacifiers and to receive no food or drink other than breast milk, unless medically indicated.

20. You have the right to be referred to a breastfeeding support group, if available, upon discharge from the birthing facility.

GLOSSARY

ACUPRESSURE: A therapy of Chinese origin that involves applying firm pressure to precise points on the skin.

ACUPUNCTURE: A therapy of Chinese origin that involves the superficial introduction of very fine needles into precise points on the skin.

ANALGESIA: General term used to denote the disappearance of perception of pain, no matter the technique used to achieve this.

AUTOGENIC (RELAXATION): Self-generated relaxation technique.

BIRTHING ROOM: Room where labor and birth take place.

BREECH PRESENTATION: Presentation of the baby where the buttocks or feet, rather than the head, will emerge from the uterus first at the time of birth.

CERVICAL EFFACEMENT: The thinning and shortening of the cervix that happens at the end of pregnancy and during labor.

CERVIX: the lower part of the uterus which opens into the vagina.

CESAREAN SECTION: Surgical intervention which involves making an incision into a pregnant woman's uterus to extract the fetus and placenta.

COMPONENTS OF PAIN:

- **Cognitive-Behavioral:** The manner in which the person expresses their experience of pain.
- **Motivational-Affective (psychological):** Allows one to judge the unpleasantness of pain.
- **Nociceptive:** Real or potential injury.
- **Sensory-Discriminative (physical):** Allows one to feel the intensity and threshold of pain.

DIASTASE OF THE RECTUS ABDOMINIS: a spacing between the rectus abdominis muscles that causes an opening of the abdominal wall. In women, it sometimes occurs after multiple pregnancies or after a pregnancy with multiples (twins, etc).

ENDORPHINS: Substances present in many structures of the central nervous system that have strong sedative and pain relieving effects.

EPIDURAL: See lumbar epidural anaesthesia.

EPISIOTOMY: Surgical cutting of the perineum designed to enlarge the opening of the vulva and facilitate the baby's exit.

FETAL MONITOR: An electronic monitor that records the electrocardiogram and cardiac frequency of the fetus and allows for the detection and possible correction of problems.

HORMONES IN LABOR:

- **Catecholamine:** hormone of excitement and stress, composed of adrenaline and noradrenaline.
- **Endorphin:** the hormone of pleasure, dependence, transcendence, and reduction of pain.
- **Oxytocin:** the hormone of love, attachment, and well-being.
- **Prolactin:** maternal milk production hormone and mothering hormone.

HYPERTENSION: Increased resting blood pressure.

HYPERVENTILATION: Abnormally deep or fast breathing caused by anxiety. Hyperventilating causes an abnormal level of CO_2 in the blood.

LABOR: The process that allows for the ejection of the baby from the uterus.

LUMBAR EPIDURAL ANAESTHESIA: method of local anesthesia, used during labor or cesarean, which aims to reduce painful sensations related to birth.

MENTAL IMAGING: the activity of producing mental images.

MERIDIAN: the trajectory of circulation of energy in the body, used in acupuncture and acupressure. The meridians form a network that connects the different internal and external elements of the body and regularizes the functioning of the organism as a whole.

OCCIPUT ANTERIOR: Position of the baby in mother's belly: the top of the baby's head is pointing downward, and its back is facing the front of the mother's stomach.

OCCIPUT POSTERIOR: Position of the baby in mother's belly: the top of the baby's head is pointing downward, and its back is facing the mother's back.

PAIN: An unpleasant sensory and emotional experience resulting from a real or potential injury. Pain is a subjective experience associated with our perception of the event and influenced by our past experiences.

PAIN MODULATION: Variation or change of pain due to different physical, psychological or pharmacological procedures.

Passing of baby gel or mucus plug: A precursory sign of labor. The loss of the baby gel is frequently accompanied by a small amount of blood originating from exposed capillaries of the cervix.

Pelvic floor: The group of muscles that cover the floor of the lesser pelvis.

Perineum: In women, a triangle of fibro-muscular tissues situated between the vagina and anus; in men, between the scrotum and the anus.

Pharmacological (intervention): an intervention requiring the use of chemical or drug medication.

Physiological birth: Birth that respects and relies on the internal functions particular to the organism.

Placenta: The organ that connects the fetus to the uterine wall and allows for the exchange of CO_2 and nutrients.

Reflex zone: A cutaneous zone, the stimulation of which, even light, initiates local and nearby pains.

Relaxin: A hormone released by the corpus luteum which makes the pelvic bone supple.

Rush: A tightening and shortening of the uterine muscles during labor, which contributes to the descent of the fetus.

Sedative: A (sometimes pharmacological) product that keeps a person awake, yet very calm.

Uterus: A hollow, muscular organ in which the fertilized egg implants, and where the growing fetus is nourished until birth.

Vagina: musculo-membraneous tube that connects the external genital organs to the uterus.

Visualization: The perception of an image created by the will as an objective visual sensation.

Vulva: The set of a woman's external genital organs.

ACKNOWLEDGEMENTS

With all my heart, I would like to thank Liette Mercier, of Les Éditions de l'Homme, who, through her judicious advice, made this work more precise and accurate. Thanks to Megan Millward and Camalo Gaskin for their meticulous work in adapting my work to English.

Thank you to my research colleagues for the hours of discussion and reflection: Dr. Guy-Paul Gagné, Nils Chaillet, PhD, Serge Marchand, PhD, Dr. Christine Gagnon, Emmanuelle Hébert, Raymond Gagnon, Malika Morisset Bonapace, Dr Kathy Bonapace, Lawrence Thériault, Sylvaine Suire, Verena Schmid, Dr Sarah Buckley, Louise Lettstrom-Hannant, Lise Bélanger, and Isabelle Lavoie.

Thank you to my professors, Pierre Leblond, Donna Fornelli, Suzanne Dupuis-Dubois, Michel Guay, Jean Lévesque, Marie-Josée Colibeau, Dolorès Cayouette, and Michelle Bouchard.

Finally, a big thank-you to my collaborators, Christine Gervais, Joanne Steben, Yves Morriset, Jacques Charest, Pierrette Lapointe, Gérald Hétu, Jean Desbiens, the students that I train around the world, the trainers, and, most of all, the parents who allow me to accompany them in their preparations for the birth of their families. I express to all of you my gratitude and recognition.

NOTES AND REFERENCES

Notes from the preface

1. Wente, A.S., and S.B. Crockenberg, «Transition to fatherhood: Lamaze preparation, adjustment difficulty and the husband-wife relationship», *Family Coordinator,* October 1976, p. 315-357.
2. Weaver, R.H., and M.S. Cranley, «An exploration of paternal-fetal attachment behavior», *Nursing Research,* vol. 32, n° 2, 1983, p. 68-72.
3. Markman, H. J., and F. S. Kadushin, «Preventive effects of Lamaze training for first-time parents: A short-term longitudinal study», *Journal of Consulting and Clinical Psychology,* vol. 54, n° 6, 1986, p. 872-874.

Notes from chapter 1

4. Poses are taken from the following works: Iyengar, G.S., *Yoga: Joyau de la femme,* Éditions Buchet/Chastel, Paris, 1990, p. 265 and following; Iyengar, G.S., Keller, R., and K. Khattab, *Yoga for Motherhood: Safe Practice for Expectant & New Mothers,* Sterling Publishing Co., New York, 2010, 443 pages.
5. There are many Iyengar yoga centers around the world, whose trainers all make use of the methodology developed by Mr. Iyengar. If you cannot find an Iyengar center, prenatal yoga is another excellent option for motivation and guidance in your practice.
6. Chuntharapat, S., Petpichetchian, W., and U. Hatthakit, «Yoga during pregnancy: Effects on maternal comfort, labor pain and birth outcomes», *Complementary Therapies in Clinical Practice,* vol. 14, n° 2, 2008, p. 105-115.
7. Shamanthakamani, N., Raghuram, N., Vivek, N., Sulochana, G., and N. Hongasandra Rama, «Efficacy of Yoga on Pregnancy Outcome», *The Journal of Alternative and Complementary Medicine,* vol. 11, n° 2, 2005, p. 237-244.
8. Cité dans Svenson, D., *Ashtanga Yoga: The practice manual,* Ashtanga Yoga Productions, Austin, Texas, 2008, p. 249.
9. Dumoulin, C., *Avant et après bébé: Exercices et conseils,* Montréal, Éditions du CHU Sainte-Justine, 2011, p. 92.
10. Rudnicki, M., Frölich, A., Rasmussen, W.F., and P. McNair, «The effect of magnesium on maternal blood pressure in pregnancy-induced hypertension: A randomized double-blind placebo-controlled trial», *Acta Obstetricia et Gynecologica Scandinavica,* vol. 70, n° 6, 1991, p. 445-450.
11. Dahle, L.O., Berg, G., Hammar, M., Hurtig, M., and L. Larsson, «The effect of oral magnesium substitution on pregnancy-induced leg

cramps», *American Journal of Obstetrics and Gynecology,* July 1995, vol. 173, n° 1, p. 175-80.

12. Makrides M, Crosby DD, Bain E, Crowther CA. «Magnesium supplementation in pregnancy», *Cochrane Database of Systematic Reviews 4,* 2014.

13. Chenard, J.-R., Charest, J., and B. Lavignolle, *Lombalgie: Dix étapes sur les chemins de la guérison,* École interactionnelle du dos, Masson, Paris, 1991, 375 pages.

14. Miller, J.M., Ashton-Miller, J.A., and J.O.L. DeLancey, «A pelvic muscle precontraction can reduce cough-related urine loss in selected women with mild SUI», *Journal of the American Geriatric Society,* n° 46, 1998, p. 870-874.

15. Carrière, B., *The pelvic floor,* Stuttgart, Georg Thieme Verlag, 2006.

16. This exercise was developed by the French midwife Sylvaine Suire.

17. Beckmann, M.M., and O.M. Stock, «Antenatal perineal massage for reducing perineal trauma», *Cochrane Database of Systematic Reviews 4,* 2013, Art. No: CD005123. DOI: 10.1002/14651858.CD005123.pub3.

18. The meta-analysis by Beckmann cited above shows a reduction in perineal lesions even when the massage is performed twice a week starting at the thirty-fifth week.

19. Stremler, R., Hodnett, E., Petryshen, P., Stevens, B., Weston, J., and A.R. Willan, «Randomized Controlled Trial of Hands-and-Knees Positioning for Occipitoposterior Position in Labor», *Birth,* n° 32, 2005, p. 243-251.

20. Kenfack, B., Ateudjieu, B., Fouelifack Ymele, F., Tebeu, P.M., Dohbit, J.S., and R.E. Mbu, «Does the Advice to Assume the Knee-Chest Position at the 36th to 37th Weeks of Gestation Reduce the Incidence of Breech Presentation at Delivery?», *Clinics in Mother and Child Health,* n° 9, 2012, 5 pages.

21. Chenia, F., and C.A. Crowther, «Does advice to assume the knee-chest position reduce the incidence of breech presentation at delivery: A randomized clinical trial», *Birth,* n° 14, 1987, p. 75-78.

Notes from chapter 2

22. Price, D.D., Harkins, S.W., and C. Baker, «Sensory-affective relationships among different types of clinical and experimental pain», *Pain,* n° 28, 1987, p. 297-307.

23. Lindblom, U., Merskey, H., Mumford, J.-M., Nathan, P.W., Noordenbos, W., and S. Sunderland, «Pain terms: A current list with definitions and notes on usage», in H. Merskey, *Classification of chronic pain: description of chronic pain syndromes and definitions of pain terms,* Amsterdam, Elsevier, 1986, p. s215-s221.

24. Odent, M., «The fetus ejection reflex», *Birth,* n° 14, 1987, p. 104-105.

25. Verera Scmid, in her book *Birth Pain: Explaining Sensations, Exploring Possibilities* (2nd ed., 2011) presents a lucid look at the role that pain plays in birth.

26. Bonica, J., «Labor pain», in P.D. Wall and R. Melzack, *Textbook of pain,* New York, Churchill Livingstone, 1994, p. 615-641.

27. Nettelbladt, P., Fagerström, C.F., and N. Uddenberg, «The significance of reported childbirth pain», *Journal of Psychosomatic Research,* n° 20, 1976, p. 215-221.

28. Norr, K.L., Block, C.R., Charles, A., Meyering, S., and E. Meyer, «Explaining pain and enjoyment in childbirth», *Journal of Health and Social Behavior,* n° 18, 1977, p. 260-275.

29. Lowe, N. K., «Explaining the pain of active labor: The importance of maternal confidence», *Research in Nursing & Health,* n° 12, 1989, p. 237-245.

30. Lowe, N.K., «The nature of labor pain», *American Journal Obstetrics and Gynecology,* n° 186, 2002, p. 16-24.

31. A *doula,* or birth companion, is a person specially experienced to support women and their partners during labor and birth. She helps the parents use non-pharmacological comfort measures, and may support them before, during, and after the birth.

32. Hodnett, E.D., Gates, S., Hofmeyr, G.J., Sakala, C., and J. Weston, «Continuous support

for women during childbirth», *Cochrane Database of Systematic Reviews 2,* 2011.

33. Hodnett, E.D., «Pain and women's satisfaction with the experience of childbirth: A systematic review», *American Journal of Obstetrics & Gynecology,* vol. 186, n° 5, Suppl. Nature, 2002, p. 160-172.

34. Leap, N., Dodwell, M., and M. Newburn, «Working with pain in labor: An overview of evidence», *New Digest,* n° 49, 2010, p. 22-26.

35. Brownridge, P., «The nature and consequences of childbirth pain», *European Journal of Obstetrics & Gynecology and Reproductive Biology,* n° 59, Suppl., 1995, p. S9-S15.

36. Alehagen, S., Wijma, B., Lundberg, U., and K. Wijma, «Fear, pain and stress hormones during childbirth», *Journal of Psychosomatic Obstetrics & Gynecology,* n° 26, 2005, p. 153-165.

37. Mahomed, K., Gulmezoglu, A.M., Nikodem, V.C., Wolman, W.L., Chalmers, B.E., and G.J. Hofmeyr, «Labor experience, maternal mood and cortisol and catecholamine levels in low-risk primiparous women», *Journal of Psychosomatic Obstetrics & Gynecology,* vol. 16, n° 4, 1995, p. 181-186.

38. Lowe, Nancy K., «The nature of labor pain», *American Journal of Obstetrics and Gynecology,* vol. 186, n° 5, 2002, p. 16-24.

39. Marchand, S., *Le phénomène de la douleur,* 2ⁿᵈ ed., Montréal, Chenelière Éducation, 2009, p. 378.

40. Price, D.D., Barrell, J.-J., and R.H. Gracely, «A psychophysical analysis of experimental factors that selectively influence the effective dimension of pain», *Pain,* n° 8, 1980, p. 137-149.

41. Price, D.D., Harkins, S.W., and C. Baker, «Sensory-affective relationships among different types of clinical and experimental pain», *Pain,* n° 28, 1987, p. 297-307.

42. Visual analog scales graded from 0 to 100 that measure the intensity and unpleasant aspect of pain allow us to better understand the experience of pain. During birth, it is preferable not to have the pain evaluated, but sometimes the evaluation may help to reassure those who are supporting the laboring woman.

43. Marchand, S., *Le phénomène de la douleur,* 2ⁿᵈ ed., Montréal, Chenelière Éducation, 2009, p. 378.

44. Jones, L., Othman, M., Dowswell, T., Alfirevic, Z., Gates, S., Newburn, M., Jordan, S., Lavender, T., and J.P., Neilson, «Pain management for women in labor: An overview of systematic reviews», *Cochrane Database of Systematic Reviews 3,* 2012.

45. Melzack, R., and P. D. Wall, «Pain mechanisms: A new theory», *Science,* n° 150, 1965, p. 971-979.

46. Ohlsson, G., Buchhave, P., Leandersson, U., Nordstrom, L., Rydhstrom, H., and I. Sjolin, «Warm tub bathing during labor: Maternal and neonatal effects», *Acta Obstetricia et Gynecologica Scandinavica,* n° 80, 2001, p. 311-314.

47. Garland, D., *Revisiting Waterbirth: An Attitude to Care,* 3ʳᵈ ed., Basingstoke, Palgrave Macmillan, 2011, 217 pages.

48. Cluett, E.R., and E. Burns, «Immersion in water in labor and birth», *Cochrane Database of Systematic Reviews 2,* 2009.

49. Roberts, J., «Maternal position during the first stage of labor», in Chalmers, I., Enkin, M., and M.J.N.C. Keirse, *Effective care in pregnancy and childbirth,* Oxford University Press, 1989, p. 883-892.

50. Roberts, J. E., Mendez-Bauer, C., and D.A. Wodell, «The effects of maternal position on uterine contractility and efficiency», *Birth,* vol. 10, n° 4, 1983, p. 243-249.

51. Lawrence, A., Lewis, L., Hofmeyr, G.J., Dowswell, T., and C. Styles, «Maternal positions and mobility during first stage labor», *Cochrane Database of Systematic Reviews 2,* 2009.

52. Gupta, J.K., Hofmeyr, G.J., and M. Shehmar, «Position in the second stage of labor for women without epidural anaesthesia», *Cochrane Database of Systematic Reviews 5,* 2012.

53. Kane, K., and A. Taub, «A history of local electrical analgesia», *Pain,* n° 1, 1975, p. 125-138.

54. Tyler, E., Caldwell, C., and J. N. Ghia, «Transcutaneous electrical nerve stimulation: An alternative approach to the management of postoperative pain», *Anesthesia and analgesia,* vol. 61, n° 5, 1982, p. 449-456.

55. Le Bars, D., Dickenson, A. H., and J.-M. Besson, «Diffuse Noxious Inhibitory Controls (DNIC) I: Effects on dorsal horn convergent neurones in the rat», *Pain,* n° 6, 1979a, p. 283-304.

56. Le Bars, D., Dickenson, A. H., and J.-M. Besson, «Diffuse Noxious Inhibitory Controls (DNIC) II: Lack of effect on non-convergent neurones, supraspinal involvement and theoretical implications», *Pain,* n° 6, 1979b, p. 305-327.

57. Smith, C.A., Collins, C.T., Crowther, C.A., and K.M. Levett, «Acupuncture or acupressure for pain management in labor», *Cochrane Database of Systematic Reviews 7,* 2011.

58. Smith, C.A., Levett, K.M., Collins, C.T., and L. Jones, «Massage, reflexology and other manual methods for pain management in labor», *Cochrane Database of Systematic Reviews 2,* 2012.

59. Smith, C.A., Collins, C.T., Crowther, C.A., and K.M., Levett, «Acupuncture or acupressure for pain management in labor», *Cochrane Database of Systematic Reviews 7,* 2011.

60. Mårtensson, L., and G., Wallin, «Sterile water injections as treatment for low back pain during labor: A review», *Australian and New Zealand journal of obstetrics and gynaecology,* vol. 48, n° 4, 2008, p. 369-374.

61. Hodnett, E.D., Gates, S., Hofmeyr, G.J., Sakala, C., and J. Weston, «Continuous support for women during childbirth», *Cochrane Database of Systematic Reviews 2,* 2011.

62. Chuntharapat, S., Petpichetchian, W. and U. Hatthakit, «Yoga during pregnancy: Effects on maternal comfort, labor pain and birth outcomes», *Complementary Therapies in Clinical Practice,* vol. 14, n° 2, 2008, p. 105-115.

63. Shamanthakamani, N., Raghuram, N., Vivek, N., Sulochana, G. and N. Hongasandra Rama, «Efficacy of Yoga on Pregnancy Outcome», *The Journal of Alternative and Complementary Medicine,* vol. 11, n° 2, 2005, p. 237-244.

64. Smith, C.A., Levett, K.M., Collins, C.T. and C.A. Crowther, «Relaxation techniques for pain management in labor», *Cochrane Database of Systematic Reviews 12,* 2011.

65. Marchand, S. and P. Arsenault, «Odors modulate pain perception: A gender-specific effect», *Physiology & behavior,* vol. 76, n° 2, 2002, p. 251-256.

66. Chaillet, N. Belaid, L. Crochetière, C., Roy, L., Gagné, G-P., Moutquin, J-M., Rossignol, M., Dugas, M., Wassef, M., and J. Bonapace, «A Meta-Analysis of Non-Pharmacologic Approaches for Pain Management during Labor: Toward a Paradigm Shift?», 2013 (submitted for publication).

67. Bonapace, J., Chaillet, N., Gaumond, I., Paul-Savoie, E., and S. Marchand, «Evaluation of the Bonapace Method: A specific educational intervention to reduce pain during childbirth», *Journal of Pain Research,* 2013, 6, p. 653-661.

Notes from chapter 3

68. Brabant, I., *Une naissance heureuse: Bien vivre sa grossesse et son accouchement,* 4th ed., Anjou Fides, 2013, 576 pages.

69. Buckley, S.J., «Undisturbed Birth: Mother Nature's hormonal blueprint for safety, ease and ecstasy», in *Gentle Birth, Gentle Mothering: A Doctors Guide to Natural Childbirth and Gentle Early Parenting Choices,* Celestial Arts, 2009, 348 pages.

70. Odent, M., *The function of the orgasms: The highways to transcendence,* London, Pinter and Martin Ltd, 2009, 213 pages.

71. Buckley, S.J., *Gentle Birth, Gentle Mothering: A Doctors Guide to Natural Childbirth and Gentle Early Parenting Choices,* Celestial Arts, 2009, 348 pages.

72. Matthiesen, A.S., A. B. Ransjo-Arvidson et al, «Postpartum maternal oxytocin release by newborns: effects of infant hand massage and sucking», *Birth,* vol. 28, n° 1, 2001, p. 13-19.

73. Tyzio, R., Cossart, R., Khalilov, I., Minlebaev, M., Hübner, C. A., Represa, A. and R. Khazipov, «Maternal oxytocin triggers a transient inhibitory switch in GABA signaling in the fetal brain during delivery», *Science,* n° 314, 5806, 2006, p. 1788-1792.

74. Odent, M., *The scientification of love,* London, Free Association Books, 2001.

75. Odent, M., *The function of the orgasms: The highways to transcendence*, Pinter and Martin Ltd, London, 2009, 213 pages.

76. Tyzio, R., Cossart, R., Khalilov, I., Minlebaev, M., Hübner, C. A., Represa, A. and R., Khazipov, «Maternal oxytocin triggers a transient inhibitory switch in GABA signaling in the fetal brain during delivery», *Science,* vol. 314, n° 5806, 2006, p. 1788-1792.

77. Zanardo, V., S. Nicolussi et al, «Beta-endorphin concentrations in human milk», *Journal of Pediatric Gastroenterology and Nutrition,* vol. 33, n° 2, 2001, p. 160-164.

78. Rivier, C., W. Vale et al, «Stimulation in vivo of the secretion of prolactin and growth hormone by beta-endorphin», *Endocrinology,* vol. 100, n° 1, 1977, p. 238-41.

   a. Browning, A.J., Butt, W.R., Lynch, S.S., Shakespear, R.A. and J.S. Crawford, «Maternal and cord plasma concentrations of beta-lipotrophin, beta-endorphin and gamma-lipotrophin at delivery; effect of analgesia», *British Journal of Obstetrics & Gynaecology,* vol. 90, n° 11, 1983, p. 1152-1156.

   b. Rivier, C., W. Vale et al, «Stimulation in vivo of the secretion of prolactin and growth hormone by beta-endorphin», *Endocrinology,* vol. 100, n° 1, 1977, p. 238-41.

   c. Zanardo, V., S. Nicolussi et al, «Beta-endorphin concentrations in human milk», *Journal of Pediatric Gastroenterology and Nutrition,* vol. 33, n° 2, 2001, p. 160-164.

79. Wiklund, I., Norman, M., Uvnäs-Moberg, K., Ransjö-Arvidson, A. B., and E. Andolf, «Epidural analgesia: Breast-feeding success and related factors», *Midwifery,* vol. 25, n° 2, 2009, p. 31-38.

80. Odent, M., *The fetus ejection reflex: The Nature of Birth and Breastfeeding,* Sydney, Ace Graphics, 1992, p. 29-43.

81. Lagercrantz, H., and T.A. Slotkin, «The 'stress' of being born», *Scientific American,* vol. 254, n° 4, 1986, p. 100-107.

82. Segal, S., Csavoy, A.N., and S. Datta, «The tocolytic effect of catecholamines in the gravid rat uterus», *Anesthesia & Analgesia,* vol. 87, n° 4, 1998, p. 864-869.

83. Uvnas-Moberg, K, «Physiological and psychological effects of oxytocin and prolactin in connection with motherhood with special reference to food intake and the endocrine system of the gut», *Acta Physiologica Scandinavica. Supplementum,* n° 583, 1989, p. 41-48.

84. Brabant, I., *Une naissance heureuse: Bien vivre sa grossesse et son accouchement,* 4th ed., Montréal, Fides, 2013, 576 pages.

85. Friedman, E. A., «Normal labor», dans Emanuel A. Friedman, *Labor: Clinical evaluation and management,* New York, Appleton-Century-Crofts, vol.2, 1978, p. 1-58.

86. Singata, M., Tranmer, J., and G.M.L. Gyte, «Restricting oral fluid and food intake during labor», *Cochrane Database of Systematic Reviews 1,* 2010.

87. Gaskin, I.M., *Spiritual Midwifery,* 4th ed., Book Publishing Company, 2002.

88. Odent, M., *The scientification of love,* London, Free Association Books, 2001.

89. Wieland Ladewig, P., London, M. L. and S. Brookens Olds, *Soins infirmiers: Maternité et néonatalogie,* Saint-Laurent, Éditions du Renouveau Pédagogique, 1992, 1002 pages.

90. Brabant, I., *Une naissance heureuse: Bien vivre sa grossesse et son accouchement,* 4th ed., Anjou, Fides, 2013, 576 pages.

91. Gaskin, I.M., *Spiritual Midwifery,* 4th ed., Book Publishing Company, 2002.

92. Hodnett, E.D., Gates, S., Hofmeyr, G.J., Sakala, C., and J. Weston, «Continuous support for women during childbirth», *Cochrane Database of Systematic Reviews 2, 2011.*

93. Newton, N., «The fetus ejection reflex revisited», *Birth*, vol. 14, n° 2, 1987, p. 106-108.

94. Odent, M., «The fetus ejection reflex», *Birth,* vol. 14, n° 2, 1987, p. 104-105.

95. Ferguson, J.K.W., «A study of the motility of the intact uterus at term», *Surgery, Gynecology & Obstetrics,* n° 63, 1941, p. 359-366.

96. Blanks, A.M. and S. Thornton, «The role of oxytocin in parturition», *British Journal of Obstetrics and Gynaecology,* vol. 110, n° 20, 2003, p. 46-51.

97. Odent, M., «The fetus ejection reflex», *Birth,* vol. 14, n° 2, 1987, p. 104-105.

98. Newton, N., Peeler, D., and M. Newton, «Effect of disturbance on labor: Experiment using one hundred mice with dated pregnancies», *American Journal of Obstetrics and Gynecology,* n° 8, 1986, p. 1096-1102.

99. Mercer, J.S., and D.A. Erickson-Owens, «Rethinking placental -transfusion and cord clamping issues», *Journal of Perinatal & Neonatal Nursing,* vol. 26, n° 3, July-September 2012, p. 202-217.

100. Anim-Somuah, M., Smyth, R.M.D., and L. Jones, «Epidural versus non-epidural or no analgesia in labor», *Cochrane Database of Systematic Reviews 12, 2011.*

101. Lieberman, E., and C. O'Donoghue, «Unintended effects of epidural analgesia during labor: a systematic review», *American Journal of Obstetrics and Gynecology,* vol. 5, n° 186, Supplement Nature, 2002, p. 31-68.

102. Carroll, T.G., Engelken, M., Mosier, M.C., and N. Nazir, «Epidural analgesia and severe perineal laceration in a community-based obstetric practice», *Journal of the American Board of Family Practice,* vol. 16, n° 1, 2003, p. 1-6.

103. Beilin, Y., et al, «Effect of labor epidural analgesia with and without fentanyl on infant breast-feeding: a prospective, randomized, double-blind study», *Anesthesiology,* 103, 6, 2005, p. 1211-1217.

104. Wiklund, I., Norman, M., Uvnäs-Moberg, K., Ransjö-Arvidson, A. B., and E. Andolf, «Epidural analgesia: Breast-feeding success and related factors», *Midwifery, 25,* 2, 2009, p. 31-38.

105. Browning, A. J., Butt, W.R., Lynch, S.S., Shakespear, R.A. and J.S. Crawford, «Maternal and cord plasma concentrations of beta-lipotrophin, beta-endorphin and gamma-lipotrophin at delivery; effect of analgesia», *British Journal of Obstetrics & Gynaecology,* vol. 90, n° 11, 1983, p. 1152-6.

106. Vadeboncoeur, H., *Une autre césarienne ou un AVAC? S'informer pour mieux décider,* 2nd ed., Anjou, Fides, 2012, 380 pages.

107. Brabant, I., *Une naissance heureuse: Bien vivre sa grossesse et son accouchement,* 4th ed. Fides, 2013, 576 pages.

108. Buckley, S. J., *Gentle Birth, Gentle Mothering: A Doctors Guide to Natural Childbirth and Gentle Early Parenting Choices,* Celestial Arts, 2009, 348 pages.

109. Roberts, C. L., Torvaldsen, S., Cameron, C. A., and E. Olive, «Delayed versus early pushing in women with epidural analgesia: A systematic review and meta-analysis», *British Journal of Obstetrics and Gynaecology: An International Journal of Obstetrics & Gynaecology,* vol. 111, n° 12, 2004, p. 1333-1340.

110. Hodnett, E.D., «Pain and women's satisfaction with the experience of childbirth: A systematic review», *American Journal of Obstetrics and Gynecology*, vol. 186, n° 5 Supplement Nature, 2002, p. 160-72.

111. Cronenwett, L.R., and L.L. Newmark, «Fathers' responses to childbirth», *Nursing Research,* 23, 3, 1974, p. 210-217.

112. Block, C.R., Norr, K.L., Meyering, S., Norr, J.-L., and A.G. Charles, «Husband gatekeeping in childbirth», *Family Relations,* April 1981, p. 197-204.

113. http://bonapace.com/docs/birthplan/sogc

Notes from chapter 4

114. Shamanthakamani, N., Raghuram, N., Vivek, N., Sulochana, G., and N. Hongasandra Rama, «Efficacy of Yoga on Pregnancy Outcome», *The Journal of Alternative and Complementary Medicine,* vol. 11, n° 2, 2005, p. 237-244.

115. Cottrell, Elizabeth C., and Jonathan R. Seckl, «Prenatal stress, glucocorticoids and the programming of adult disease», *Frontiers in Behavioral Neuroscience,* n° 3, 2009, p. 1-9.

116. Peper, E., and M. MacHose, «Symptom prescription: Inducing anxiety by 70% exhalation», *Biofeedback and Self Regulation,* vol. 18, n° 3, 1993, p. 133-139.

117. The sound BOA is from Elisa Benassi, Italian psychophonetician and midwife. www.esserevoce.it

Notes from chapter 5

118. Roberts, J., «Maternal position during the first stage of labor», in Chalmers, I., Enkin, M., and M.J.N.C. Keirse, *Effective care in pregnancy and childbirth,* Oxford University Press, 1989, p. 883-892.

119. Roberts, J.E., Mendez-Bauer, C., and D.A. Wodell, «The effects of maternal position on uterine contractility and efficiency», *Birth,* vol. 10, n° 4, 1983, p. 243-249.

120. Lawrence, A., Lewis, L., Hofmeyr, G.J., Dowswell, T., and C. Styles, «Maternal positions and mobility during first stage labor», *Cochrane Database of Systematic Reviews 2,* 2009.

121. Gupta, J.K., Hofmeyr, G.J., and M. Shehmar, «Position in the second stage of labor for women without epidural anaesthesia», *Cochrane Database of Systematic Reviews 5,* 2012.

122. Lawrence, A., Lewis, L., Hofmeyr, G.J., Dowswell, T., and C. Styles «Maternal positions and mobility during first stage labor», *Cochrane Database of Systematic Reviews 2,* 2009.

123. Balaskas, J., *Active birth: the new approach to giving birth naturally,* Boston, The Harvard Common Press, 1992, 252 pages.

124. Simkin, P., *The birth partner: A complete guide to childbirth for dads, doulas, and all other labor companions,* Boston, The Harvard Common Press, 2008, 398 pages.

125. Calais-Germain, B., *Bouger en accouchant: Comment le bassin peut bouger lors de l'accouchement,* Éditions DésIris, 2009, 172 pages.

126. Simkin, P., and R. Ancheta, *The labor progress handbook: Early interventions to prevent and treat dystocia,* 3rd ed., Iowa, Wiley-Blackwell, 2012, 399 pages.

127. Brabant, I., *Une naissance heureuse: Bien vivre sa grossesse et son accouchement,* 4th ed., Anjou Fides, 2013, 576 pages.

128. De Gasquet, B., *Bien-être et maternité: La grossesse, la naissance et après. Forme, détente, sérénité,* Paris, Éditions Albin Michel, 2009, 375 pages.

129. Engelmann, G., *Labor among primitive people,* 2nd ed., St-Louis, J. H. Chambers & Co., 1884, 227 pages.

130. Gaskin, I. M., *Ina May's Guide to Childbirth,* New York, Bantam Books, 2003, 348 pages.

131. Gaskin, I. M, *Spiritual Midwifery,* 4th ed., Summertown, Book Publishing Company, 2002, 481 pages.

132. Calais-Germain, B., *Bouger en accouchant: Comment le bassin peut bouger lors de l'accouchement,* Éditions DésIris, 2009, 172 pages.

133. A rebozo is a large scarf used to massage and relieve women during pregnancy and labor. This technique originated in Latin America. The rebozo can also be used to transport the baby during the first three years of life.

134. Adapted from Balaskas, J., *Active birth: the new approach to giving birth naturally,* Boston, The Harvard Common Press, 1992, p. 117.

135. Simkin, P., and R. Ancheta, *The labor progress handbook: Early interventions to prevent and treat dystocia,* 3rd éd., Iowa, Wiley-Blackwell, 2012, 399 pages.

136. Gardosi, J., Hutson, N., et C. B. Lynch, «Randomised, Controlled trial of squatting in the second stage of labor», *Lancet,* n° 2, 1989, p. 74.

137. Gupta, J.K., Hofmeyr, G.J., et M. Shehmar, «Position in the second stage of labor for women without epidural anaesthesia», *Cochrane Database of Systematic Reviews 5*, 2012.

138. The website of American midwife Gail Tully provides tools for learning numerous movements that can be practiced to promote optimal positioning of the baby in the uterus during pregnancy and birth. http://spinningbabies.com/ Last modified on 9 April, 2015.

139. Calais-Germain, B., *Le périnée féminin et l'accouchement,* Méolans-Revel, Éditions DésIris, 1996, 158 pages.

140. Yildirim, G., and N. Kizilkaya Beji, «Effects of Pushing Techniques in Birth on Mother and Fetus: A Randomized Study», *Birth,* vol. 35, n° 1, 2008, p. 25-30.

141. Gupta, J.K., Hofmeyr, G.J., and M. Shehmar, «Position in the second stage of labor for women without epidural anaesthesia», *Cochrane Database of Systematic Reviews 5,* 2012.

142. McKay, S., and J. Roberts, «Maternal position during labor and birth: What have we learned?», *International Childbirth Education Association,* vol. 13, n° 2, 1989, p. 19-30.

143. Roberts, J., and L. Hanson, «Best Practices in Second Stage Labor Care: Maternal Bearing Down and Positioning», *Midwifery Womens Health,* n° 52, 2007, p. 238-245.

144. Roberts, J., «Alternative positions for childbirth, Part 2: Second stage labor», *Journal of Nurse-Midwifery,* vol. 25, n° 5, 1980, p. 13-19.

145. Roberts, J. E., Goldstein, S. A., Gruener, J.-S., Maggio, M., and C. Mendez-Bauer, «A descriptive analysis of involuntary bearing-down efforts during the expulsive phase of labor», *Journal of Obstetric, Gynecologic & Neonatal Nursing,* n° 16, 1987, p. 48-55.

146. Sleep, J., Roberts, J., and I. Chalmers, «Care during the second stage of labor» dans Chalmers, I., Enkin, M., et M.J.N.C. Keirse, *Effective care in pregnancy and childbirth*, Oxford University Press, 1989, p. 1129-1136.

147. Engelmann, G., *Labor among primitive people,* 2nd ed., St-Louis, J. H. Chambers & Co., 1884, 227 pages.

148. Gupta, J.K., Hofmeyr, G.J., and M. Shehmar, «Position in the second stage of labor for women without epidural anaesthesia», *Cochrane Database of Systematic Reviews 5, 2012.*

149. Beynon, C. L., «The normal second stage of labor: A plea for reform in its conduct», *Journal of Obstetrics & Gynaecology of the British Empire,* vol. 64, n° 815, 1957, p. 331-333.

150. Odent, M., «The fœtus ejection reflex», *Birth,* vol. 14, n° 2, 1987, p. 104-105.

151. Blanks, A.M., and S. Thornton, «The role of oxytocin in parturition», *British Journal of Obstetrics and Gynaecology,* vol. 110, n° 20, 2003, p. 46-51.

152. Iyengar, G.S., Keller, R., and K. Khattab, *Yoga for Motherhood, Safe Practice for Expectant & New Mothers,* Sterling Publishing Co., New York, 2010, 443 pages.

153. Roberts, J., Goldstein, S., Gruener, J., Maggio, M., and C. Mendez-Bauer, «A Descriptive Analysis of Involuntary Bearing-down Efforts During the Expulsive Phase of Labor», *Journal of Obstetric, Gynecologic, & Neonatal Nursing,* janvier-février, 1987, p. 48-55.

154. Aasheim, V., Nilsen, A.B.V., Lukasse, M., and L.M. Reinar, «Perineal techniques during the second stage of labor for reducing perineal trauma», *Cochrane Database of Systematic Reviews 12,* 2011.

155. Carroli, G., and L. Mignini, «Episiotomy for vaginal birth», *Cochrane Database of Systematic Reviews 1,* 2009.

156. Beckmann, M.M., and A.J. Garrett, «Antenatal perineal massage for reducing perineal trauma», *Cochrane Database of Systematic Reviews 1,* 2006.

157. Odent, M., «The fœtus ejection reflex», *Birth,* vol. 14, n° 2, 1987, p. 104-105.

158. Newton, N., Foshee, D. and M. Newton, «Parturient mice: Effect of environment on labor», *Science,* n° 151, 1966, p. 1560-61.

159. Hastings-Tolsma, M., Vincent, D., Emeis, C., and T. Francisco, «Getting through birth in one piece: Protecting the perineum», American *Journal of Maternal Child Nursing,* vol. 32, n° 3, 2007, p. 158-164.

160. Beynon, C. L., «The normal second stage of labor: A plea for reform in its conduct», *Journal of Obstetrics & Gynaecology of the British Empire,* vol. 64, n° 815, 1957, p. 331-333.

161. Prins, M., Boxem, J., Lucas, C., and E. Hutton, «Effect of spontaneous pushing versus Valsalva pushing in the second stage of labor on mother and fetus: a systematic review of randomised trials», *British Journal of Obstetrics and Gynaecology,* 2011, p. 662-670.

162. Balaskas, Janet, *Active birth: The new approach to giving birth naturally,* Boston, The Harvard Common Press, 1992, p. 191-192.

163. http://bonapace.com/films/BirthDay

164. http://bonapace.com/films/orgasmicbirth

165. http://bonapace.com/films/birthasweknowit

Notes from chapter 6

166. Guiraud-Sobral, A., *Manuel pratique d'acupuncture en obstétrique,* Éditions DésIris, 2012, 111 pages.

167. Auteroche, B., *Acupuncture en gynécologie et obstétrique,* Paris, Éditions Maloine, 1986, 308 pages.

168. Beal, M.W., «Acupuncture and related treatment modalities, Part II: Applications to antepartal and intrapartal care», *Journal of Nurse-Midwifery,* vol. 37, n° 4, 1992, p. 260-268.

169. Rempp, C., and A. Bigler, *La pratique de l'acupuncture,* Paris, Éditions La Tisserande, 1992, 215 pages.

170. Salagnac, B., *Naissance et acupuncture,* 3rd ed., Montréal, Éditions Maisonneuve, 1998, 212 pages.

171. Lee, M.K., Chang, S.B., and D.H. Kang, «Effects of SP-6 acupressure on labor pain and length of delivery time in women during labor», *Journal of Alternative & Complementary Medicine,* vol. 10, n° 6, 2004, p. 959-965.

172. Hjelmstedt, A., Shenoy, S.T., Stener-Victorin, E., Lekander, M., Bhat, M., Balakumaran, L., and U. Waldenström, «Acupressure to reduce labor pain: a randomized controlled trial», *Acta Obstetricia et Gynecologica Scandinavica,* vol. 89, n° 11, 2010, p. 1453-1459.

173. Borup, L., Wurlitzer, W., Hedegaard, M., Kesmodel, U.S., and L. Hvidman, «Acupuncture as pain relief during delivery: A randomized controlled trial», *Birth,* vol. 36, n° 1, 2009, p. 5-12.

174. Hjelmstedt, A., Shenoy, S.T., Stener-Victorin, E., Lekander, M., Bhat, M., Balakumaran, L., and U. Waldenström, «Acupressure to reduce labor pain: A randomized controlled trial», *Acta Obstetricia et Gynecologica Scandinavica,* vol. 89, n° 11, 2010, p. 1453-1459.

Notes from chapter 7

175. Dick-Read, G.D., *Childbirth without fear: The principles and practice of natural childbirth,* New York, Harper and Brothers, 1953, 298 pages.

176. Jacobson, E., *Progressive relaxation,* University of Chicago Press, 1968, 496 pages.

177. Schultz, J.H., *Le training autogène,* Paris, Presses universitaires de France, 1968, 274 pages.

Notes from chapter 8

178. Chaillet, N., Belaid, L., Crochetière, C., Roy, L., Gagné, G.-P., Moutquin, J.-M., Rossignol, M., Dugas, M., Wassef, M., and J. Bonapace, «A Meta-Analysis of Non-Pharmacologic Approaches for Pain Management during Labor: Toward a Paradigm Shift?», 2013 (submitted for publication).

179. Klemp, H., *The spiritual exercises of Eck,* Minneapolis, Eckankar, 1993, 306 pages.

180. http://www.rogercallahan.com

181. Feinstein, D., «Acupoint stimulation in treating psychological disorders: Evidence of efficacy», *Review of General Psychology,* vol. 16, nº 4, 2012, p. 364.

182. Ortner, N., *The tapping solution: A revolutionary system for stress-free living,* California, Hay House Publishing, 2013, 229 pages.

183. http://eckankar.org

Notes from appendix 2

184. This original recipe was created by Nina Munthe-Lepage, certified nutrition educator.

185. Le groupe Fleurbec, *Plantes sauvages comestibles: Guide d'identification Fleurbec,* Le groupe Fleurbec inc., 1981, p. 111.

TABLE OF CONTENTS

Printed by Imprimerie Transcontinental, Beauceville, Canada